Berries

The Complete Guide to Cooking with
POWER-PACKED BERRIES

STEPHANIE PEDERSEN

STERLING
New York

This book is dedicated to you. Thank you.

STERLING
New York

An Imprint of Sterling Publishing Co., Inc.
1166 Avenue of the Americas
New York, NY 10036

ISBN 978-1-4549-1835-6

Distributed in Canada by Sterling Publishing Co., Inc.
C/o Canadian Manda Group, 664 Annette Street
Toronto, Ontario, Canada M6S 2C8
Distributed in the United Kingdom by GMC Distribution Services
Castle Place, 166 High Street, Lewes, East Sussex, England BN7 1XU
Distributed in Australia by Capricorn Link (Australia) Pty. Ltd.
P.O. Box 704, Windsor, NSW 2756, Australia

For information about custom editions, special sales, and premium and corporate purchases,
please contact Sterling Special Sales at 800-805-5489 or specialsales@sterlingpublishing.com.

Manufactured in Canada

2 4 6 8 10 9 7 5 3 1

www.sterlingpublishing.com

Photo Credits: All photography by Bill Milne © Sterling Publishing Co., Inc., with the following exceptions:
Depositphotos: © Alexstar: 65, © duskbabe: 91, © ewastudio: 101, © Anton Ignatenco: 92, © jianghongyan: 139,
© mateno: 169, © margo555: 147, © mvw@tut.by: 72, © John A Trax Jr: 73, © valentinar: 110, © Edd Westmacott:
167; iStockphoto: © Sezer Alcinkaya: 85, © Eduard Vulcan: 66; Shutterstock: © Aprilphoto: 123, © arhimax: v,
© bonchan: 95, © DronG: 112, © Iurii Kachkovskyi: 86, 157, © Maks Narodenko: 61, 71, 145, © Maxsol: 129,
© Nattika: 130, © Production Perig: 54, © Tim UR: 102; Stocksy: © Blai Baules: 162, © Rob Campbell: viii,
© Canan Czemmel: 2, © Goodness Grace Photography: 175, © Pavel Gramatikov: 5, © Lior Zilberstein: vi

CONTENTS

Introduction iv

CHAPTER 1: Getting Friendly with Berries 1

CHAPTER 2: All About the Berries 7

CHAPTER 3: Drink Your Berries 53

CHAPTER 4: Berries for Breakfast 75

CHAPTER 5: Berries for Lunch 89

CHAPTER 6: Berry Snacks 107

CHAPTER 7: Berries for Dinner 119

CHAPTER 8: Berries for Dessert 143

CHAPTER 9: Berry Condiments 163

CHAPTER 10: Frequently Asked Questions 175

Resources 178

About the Author 179

Acknowledgments 179

Index 181

Berries played a special role in my childhood. I grew up in a religion that required us to keep at least a one-year supply of food. To meet this requirement, our family not only kept a large kitchen garden (which featured a mammoth strawberry patch), but also foraged enthusiastically—especially berries. Each July my grandparents would drive from their home in southern Nevada to ours in northern California. We'd pack a picnic and load the station wagon with buckets, boxes, and heavy gloves and head off for the county road that ran behind the railroad tracks. After choosing a snake-free spot, safely removed from the road, all three generations would pick wild boysenberries (a variety of blackberry) until the containers were filled. Hours later—sweaty, prickly, and stained—we'd squeeze back into the car and head for home. Almost immediately upon entering the kitchen, my mother and grandmother (I helped when I was older) began the long, hot job of preserving the harvest: They'd make berry leather, jam, syrup, and even freeze whole berries in large Tupperware containers. What's so interesting about my berry story, however, is how ordinary it is. Almost everyone I know has a story about childhood berry picking—and berry eating—and even berry therapies.

The mother of one of my friends would use smashed strawberries mixed with sugar as a brightening mask. Another gathered the leaves from raspberry bushes and brewed them into a tea, which, she said, "helped with mommy problems." A college roommate always ate blackberries when she felt constipated. I've relied on various elderberry concoctions my entire life to protect against colds and flu. And most every friend I have turns immediately to unsweetened cranberry juice the moment a UTI (urinary tract infection) appears. Interestingly enough, research has been conducted on these and other berry remedies, showing that folk remedies actually do work! I'll share some of them with you in the chapters ahead.

Unlike many trendy health foods, berries are no fad food: Berries have a long and venerable history as health foods and beauty ingredients. In this book, you'll learn more about using and enjoying these berries and their heath benefits:

Acai
Blueberry (including bilberry)
Blackberry (and varieties)
Cranberry
Currant, Black
Current, Red and Elderberry
Goji berry

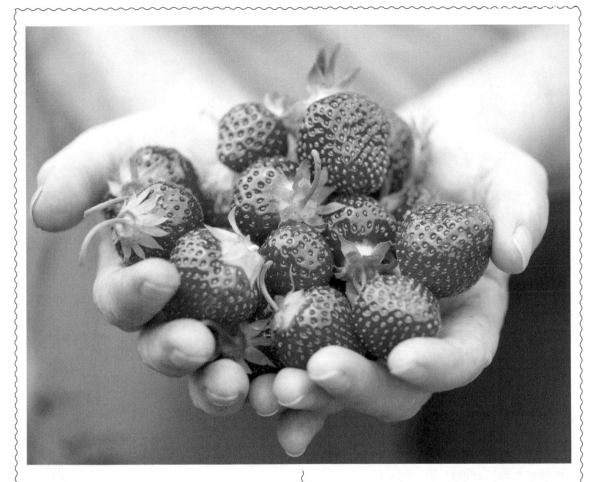

Gooseberry
Lingonberry
Mulberry
Raspberry
Sea buckthorn
Strawberry
Sweet, tart, juicy, sensual, and healthy, berries are universally loved. In fact, consumption of all berry varieties is higher than ever. Take blueberries, for instance: In the United States in 1997, the average adult consumed about 13 ounces (370g) of blueberries per year. Ten years later, in 2007, that amount nearly doubled and reached an average of 22 ounces (625 g) per year. In 2015, consumption of blueberries has nearly doubled the average for 2007. Canada, Europe, and South America have shown

similar jumps in blueberry consumption. It's not just blueberries that the world loves. European—and Russian—imports of fresh cranberries from the United States increased by 40 percent between 2012 and 2013.

Greater demand for berries globally also explains why more and more food companies are widening their distribution in order to supply consumers with snacks that include berries. Many nutritionists name cranberry, blueberry, mulberry, goji berry, or another of the world's more than 100 edible berries, as their favorite superfood. According to menu research from Datassential (a data tracking and collecting company), the inclusion of berries on menus has "greatly increased" every year since 2011. Entire blogs are devoted to berries. Supplements derived from cranberry, mulberry, blueberry, and other berries have outsold all other types of botanical-based supplements since 2011. And research studies of berries, and their effects on health, are at an all-time high.

Clearly, people are interested in knowing more about how to use this important superfood to maintain their health, and no wonder: Berries have been shown to have a positive impact on conditions as far ranging as cardiovascular disease, arthritis, dementia, diabetes, and cancer. And because berries are lower in sugars than most fruits, they have become a staple with the paleo, vegan,

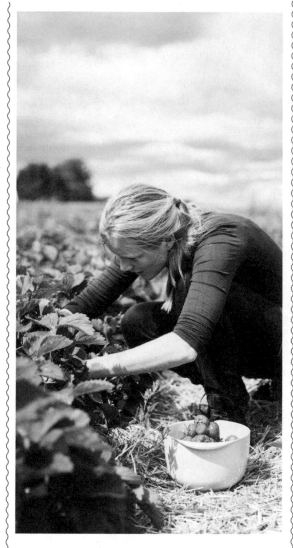

and raw-food crowd. Just as significantly, berries are often one of the only plant foods that frustrated moms can get their children (and husbands) to eat. Berries of all kinds, and in various forms (dried, freeze-dried, frozen, and fresh), have even found a place among mainstream foodies looking for a convenient, flavorful way to add nourishing fiber, vitamins, powerful antioxidants, and a large range of healing phytonutrients to their diets.

Part of the growing popularity of berries has to do with "the berry evangelists"— celebrity doctors, for example, who list one or more types of berries as must-have components of a healthful diet. More than ever, food bloggers, health counselors, and nutritionists are encouraging people to increase their berry intake. And various berry growers in the United States and elsewhere spend more than $60 million a year to not only educate consumers about berries and their benefits but also to help spread the good news to all of us. That means in-depth health education, recipe guides, and more.

Perhaps you noticed strawberries being touted as a cholesterol-lowering food on several news programs? Or blueberries in a book on brain health? Or mulberries on a talk-show host's television show and website? Teaching us how to choose and use berries to stay healthy is a big-buck business. Which, in my book, is just fine. In my eyes, anything that is going to help you get and stay healthy is worth spending money on. And there's so much more, all of which I'll share in the chapters ahead.

But health benefits aside, people simply like the sweet-tart and highly addictive (in a healthy way!) flavor of berries. So maybe it's not so surprising that fresh berries are one of America's most frequently consumed snack foods, or that Produce For Better Health Foundation's *State of the Plate 2014* reports that among all age ranges, berries of all kinds are the third most frequently consumed fruit in the United States (behind bananas and apples). Unlike stronger-tasting superfoods, such as Brussels sprouts or kale, berries are not an acquired taste: Most people already love them! Also unlike other powerfoods—including broccoli, chia, and salmon—berries are convenient. No need to do any peeling or chopping—just give them a quick rinse and enjoy.

But don't stop there. Berries deserve a starring role in each of your meals! In this book, I show you how to enjoy these lovely fruits in juices, smoothies, and cocktails; frozen treats (like popsicles made from pureed berries, unsweetened coconut water or coconut milk, and a few chia seeds); baked goods, desserts, candy, and other snack foods; fruit and green salads; grain dishes; and even as dried fruit and fruit leather. Berries add a delicious pop of flavor and a host of nutrients wherever (and however) they are enjoyed. I can't wait to show you more ways to use these versatile and delicious ingredients!

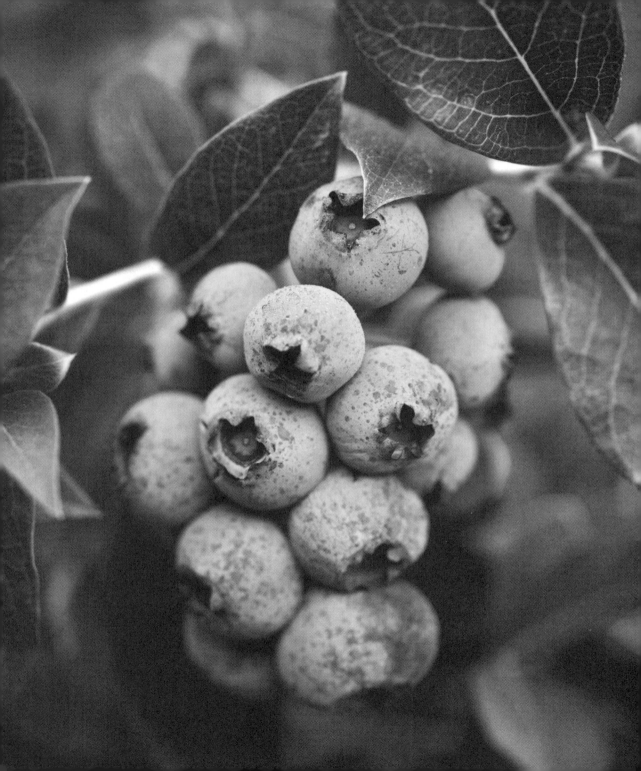

CHAPTER 1

GETTING FRIENDLY WITH BERRIES

Hello, berry lovers! I am so excited to share one of my favorite superfruits with you as well as to welcome all of you who are looking for delicious ways to improve your health and make sure your loved ones get the nutrition they need to be their best.

Before I go any further, let's talk about the word *berry*. In botanical terms, *berry* refers to a fruit with an edible fleshy portion (known as the pericarp), and which develops from the ovary of a single flower. This means bananas, cucumbers, eggplants, and tomatoes are all "berries"—and strawberries and raspberries are not. I have chosen to ignore science, however—at least in this instance (but there will be plenty of it in the pages to come!)—and use the definition that is most familiar to us: A berry is a small, pulpy and often edible fruit. In *Berries: The Complete Guide to Cooking With Power-Packed Berries*, the focus is on edible berries, including acai, blueberries (and it's wild sibling, bilberries), blackberries (with all its varieties), cranberries, fresh currants (both black and red), elderberries, goji berries, gooseberries, hawthorn, lingonberries, mulberries (standard and white), raspberries (red and yellow), and strawberries.

Anthropologists believe that berries were one of humankind's earliest foods, prized as much for their bright flavor as their ability to help early humans feel their best. Ancient Greeks used many different berries to treat myriad conditions, from diarrhea to anemia. Berries of several kinds, including blackberries, were described as cures in the ancient Byzantine medical text, *Juliana Anicia Codex*, a richly illustrated manuscript that was presented as a gift to Princess Juliana Anicia of Constantinople in 512 CE.

Across the Atlantic, early North American people were using their local berries in a variety of important ways. For instance, many North American groups used raspberries (as well as the leaves) to help strengthen the uterus for pregnancy. In the 1600s and 1700s, cranberries were used to prevent wintertime scurvy among pilgrims and other settlers in North America. In the 1800s, hawthorn berries were commonly

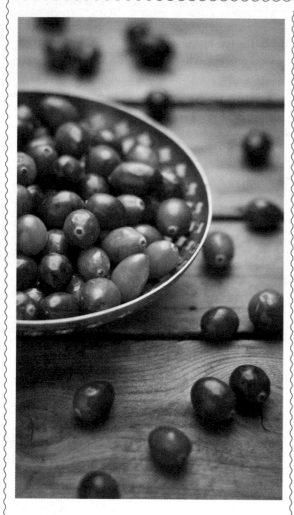

Soon, studies were organized to learn just what berries can and cannot do.

As the public began to learn more about nutrients—and what foods contained what nutrients—interest in berries grew. Individuals could use vitamin-rich berries to easily keep themselves and their families healthy and prevent illnesses that would require expensive doctor's visits and pricey medicine to treat.

In the world of late nineteenth century to early twentieth century agriculture, something else was happening that also elevated the status of berries. Individual berry growers began to band together and form grower's associations. One of the oldest of these is the Cape Cod Cranberry Growers Association, established in 1888. Others, such as the current MBG, which began in 1936 as the Michigan Blueberry Growers Association, has since expanded to include berry growers from across the United States and Canada. By the 1940s there were hundreds of berry grower's associations around the world, most of which boasted marketing departments that helped initiate a groundswell of consumer interest in their products. To incite even greater interest in berries, marketers began to publicize the growing number of health studies that were being conducted and that touted the health benefits of berries. Soon, women's magazines

prescribed to treat circulatory disorders and respiratory conditions. In the first two decades of the 1900s, researchers began discovering vitamins, minerals, and other nutrients, allowing the medical community to conduct research into exactly what it is about berries that makes them so healthful.

got involved, publishing health-oriented articles and tantalizing berry recipes, which lured home cooks into the marketplace and into the kitchen.

Since then, our love affair with this beautiful superfruit has only grown stronger. All you have to do is hop onto the Internet or pick up one of dozens of magazines to find stories touting the disease-fighting power of these miniature fruits. Television news segments routinely reference scientific studies that credit blackberries, cranberries, strawberries, and increasingly, "superfood" berries such as acai, goji, and blueberries for conferring multiple health benefits—

from lowering one's chance of developing cancer to clearing urinary tract infections to improving eyesight and much more. From my own experience, I have found that a daily berry habit helps keep my energy level high and my immune system strong—especially important in the dark days of cold and flu season, when I get sneezed on every time I venture onto New York City sidewalks and my children come home sick from school.

How did berries get so trendy? The fact that they taste amazing doesn't hurt their star power, but it's their disease-fighting properties that have made them so popular. An example of this is that Great Britain produced about 300 tons of blueberries a year until 2010, when research studies about the antioxidant power of blueberries began circulating in the British media. By 2013, production had rocketed to 1,747 tons. According to Nielsen Perishables Group, which tracks sales of fresh fruit at grocery stores, in 2013, consumers in the United States bought more than $3 billion of different types of berries, from raspberries to gooseberries to blackberries and more.

While each of the berries celebrated in this book has a different nutrient profile that provides a unique combination of healing benefits, all of them are worthy additions to your daily diet. And because there is a berry for almost every season—from strawberries in spring to blackberries in summer and cranberries in autumn—it is easy to enjoy them every day of the year. In fact, developing a daily berry habit, as I tell all of my clients, is an easy way to reduce inflammation, ward off a host of health conditions, and even help treat a health condition you may currently be up against.

As you peruse the pages of this book, be prepared to discover new berry varieties as well as rediscover old favorites. You'll learn more about their nutrient content and have an opportunity to experiment with delicious, whole food, superfood recipes. And although it's true that berries taste great eaten out of

BERRIES' ANCIENT ORIGINS

Berries of all varieties, whether they grow on bushes, trees, or the ground, have been prized as food since the beginning of time—and not only for humans and prehumans: Bears, monkeys, birds, deer, and other animals have relied, and continue to rely, on berries for a large portion of their diet.

Early humans, wanting to enjoy wild berries long after the last one had been plucked from its bramble, quickly learned that drying a portion of their harvest—either as whole berries, or in the form of paste—was an easy, delicious way to enjoy the fruit's sweet-tart flavor and disease-fighting power year-round.

Tired of competing with birds and bears for their berries, people began growing their own fruit around the fourth century CE. At about the same time, written instructions for cultivating berries (specifically raspberries) began to appear, many of them written by Roman agriculturist Palladius.

hand or tossed here and there on yogurt and cereal, there is so, so much more you can do with them. Having lots of recipes for many different types of berries is a great way to make sure you get all the benefits of these nutrition powerhouses into your diet every day. Ready to learn more? Turn the page!

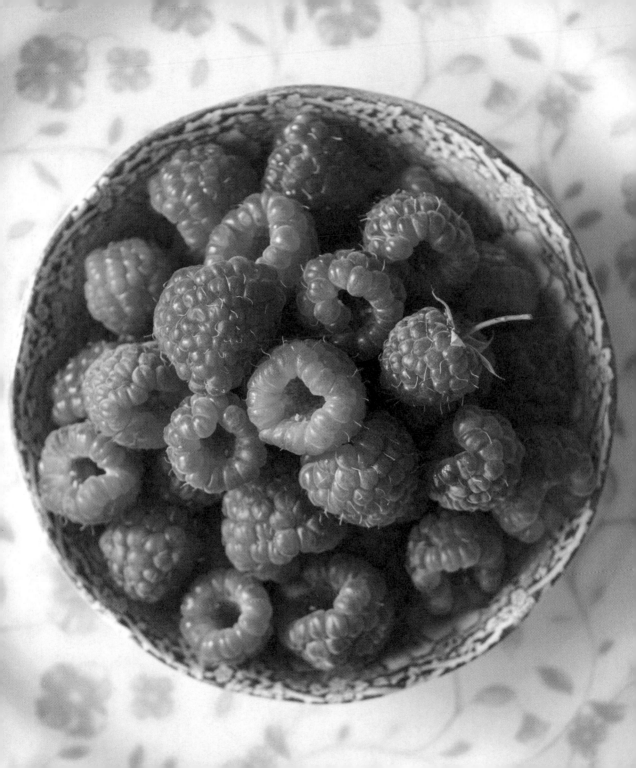

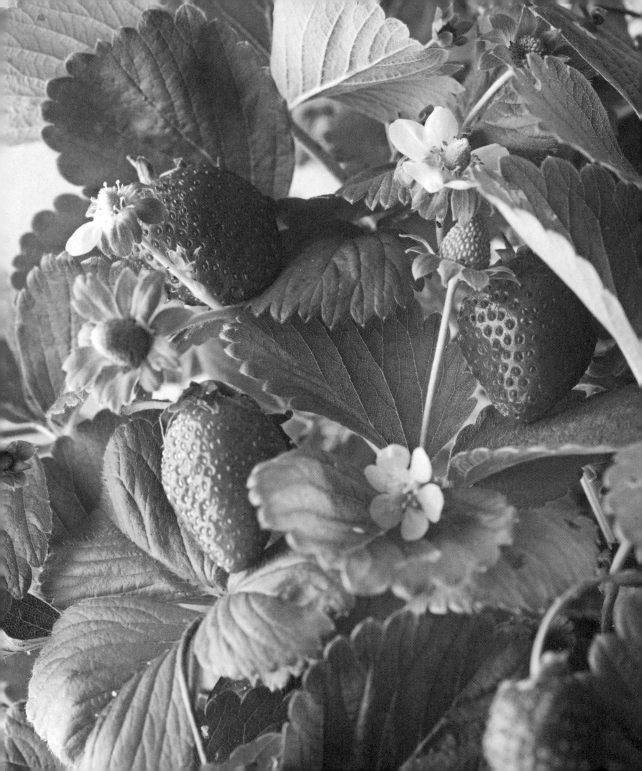

CHAPTER 2

ALL ABOUT
THE BERRIES

Berries may be one of the most well-loved superfoods around. Just think about it: Do you know anyone who doesn't like at least one type of berry? These small, delicious fruits come in a wide range of styles—from orb-shaped currants, blueberries, and cranberries to soft, fleshy raspberries and blackberries, to heart-shaped strawberries—each with slightly different uses, flavors, and nutritional strengths. This is a good thing: Our bodies love variety, and enjoying a number of these lovely fruits allows your body to get a wide range of health-supportive nutrients. That's why I encourage my clients to enjoy at least two or three servings of berries each week. And by berries, I mean the fruits known as culinary berries—even though, botanically, some belong to other plant families.

In my household, we enjoy fresh berries when they are in season—from late-autumn cranberries to spring strawberries to summer raspberries. Year-round, we toss fresh or frozen berries into smoothies, baked goods, sauces, relishes, dips, and a wide variety of both sweet and savory dishes for just about every meal, treat, and snack of the day. This makes it easy for us to get the high levels of phytonutrients, fiber, and vitamins A, B complex, C, E, and K, as well as minerals, such as manganese, that berries provide. These nutrients help us ward off viruses during cold and flu season, keep our skin looking good all year, help prevent cancer, protect our eyesight, support nervous-system health, help treat urinary tract infections (UTIs), improve our cardiovascular system, and so much more—all with lower sugar levels than many fruits.

This chapter is meant to give you as much information as possible about the wide range of berries that are featured in the recipe section of this book and the astonishing things they can do, not only to improve your health and well-being, but also to bring delicious flavors and textures to every meal of the day as well. Here, you'll learn about the nutritional profile and health benefits of each berry and where it comes from, as well as how to choose and store it. I'll also suggest tips and tricks for using each berry successfully.

ACAI *(pronounced ah-sigh-EE)*

NUTRITION PROFILE

PER SERVING:

(⅜ cup/3.5 ounces/100 g acai pulp)

BACKGROUND: Acai is a deep purple South American berry that looks a bit like a small blueberry—except only 17 percent of the berry is fruit. The other 83 percent is seed. Its almost perfect essential amino acid complex, in conjunction with antioxidants and valuable trace minerals, makes acai helpful for proper muscle contraction and regeneration. Calories and nutrients can differ depending upon how, where, and in what climate the fruit is grown as well as how long it travels to reach you. Because acai berries are so very fragile, they are pureed into pulp (usually sold in 3.5-ounce pouches), juiced, frozen, dried, or made into powder immediately after harvest.

CALORIES: 150

FIBER: A serving of acai provides 3 g of fiber, which helps promote digestive health and a feeling of fullness, so you eat less. Fiber has been found to lower the risk of colorectal cancer and other gastrointestinal cancers.

PROTEIN: At 2 g of protein per serving, acai pulp has a respectable amount of protein, the macronutrients responsible for helping your body repair itself.

OMEGA-3 FATTY ACIDS: A serving of acai pulp provides 625 mcg of omega-3 fatty acids, a nutrient that reduces inflammation and may help lower the risk of chronic diseases such as heart disease, cancer, and arthritis. Symptoms of omega-3 fatty acid deficiency include fatigue, poor memory, heart problems, and mood swings.

VITAMIN A: This important vitamin supports cell growth and plays an essential role in the normal formation and maintenance of the heart, lungs, kidneys, and other organs. A serving of acai pulp will give you 750 international units (IUs) of vitamin A.

VITAMIN B_6: The body uses vitamin B_6 for more than 100 enzyme reactions involved in metabolism as well as brain development and immune function in utero and during infancy. A serving of acai pulp will give you about 0.052 mg—or 4 percent of the recommended daily intake of 1.3 mg—of vitamin B_6.

VITAMIN C: This powerful antioxidant can help prevent and lessen the duration of vital illnesses, stimulate collagen production for fast wound healing, and help prevent a variety of diseases, from cancer to cataracts. A serving of acai pulp will provide 4.8 mg of vitamin C.

AMINO ACIDS: Amino acids are the building blocks of protein. Acai berries contain nineteen different amino acids. Regular consumption of amino acids strengthens the immune system and helps the body fight infections and disease.

CALCIUM: In addition to its well-known role as a bone-and-teeth builder, calcium helps the body's muscles move and enables nerves to carry messages between the brain and other parts of the body. Acai pulp provides 20 g of calcium per serving.

COPPER: Low copper intake has been associated with high cholesterol and cardiovascular disease in some individuals. Acai provides 0.2 mg of copper per serving.

IRON: In addition to its role in red-blood-cell production, iron is necessary for growth, normal cell function, and synthesis of some

hormones and connective tissues. Acai provides 2 mg of this important mineral.

MANGANESE: This essential nutrient is involved in many chemical interactions in the body, including processing cholesterol, carbohydrates, and protein. While no dietary allowance of manganese has been established by the USDA, or any other organization, 1.0 to 7.5 mg is considered an adequate daily dosage. Acai contains approximately 3 mg manganese per serving.

MAGNESIUM: More than 300 biochemical reactions in the body require magnesium. The nutrient helps maintain normal nerve and muscle function, supports a healthy immune system, keeps the heartbeat steady, and helps bones remain strong. A serving of acai pulp provides approximately 24 mg.

PHOSPHORUS: This mineral makes up 1 percent of the body's total weight. It is present in every cell of the body—particularly in bones and teeth. A serving of acai provides about 14 mg.

POTASSIUM: This mineral is crucial to body functions. 3.5 ounces of acai pulp provides 135 mg of the RDA.

RIBOFLAVIN: Our bodies use riboflavin (aka vitamin B_2) to break down carbohydrates, proteins, and fats and to help the body use oxygen. A serving of acai provides 0.056 mg of this nutrient.

RDA, USDA, AND YOU

In the United States, you often read about RDAs—recommended dietary allowances. The US Department of Agriculture (USDA) assigns an RDA to most nutrients. This number represents the ideal average daily intake of the nutrients. You'll find this number referred to as *RDA, recommended dietary allowance,* or *daily requirement.* The three terms are used interchangeably throughout this book.

THIAMINE: Also known as vitamin B_1, thiamine helps the body's cells change carbohydrates into energy. Small amounts of thiamine are found in most foods, including acai, a serving of which contains 0.048 mg.

ZINC: Found in cells throughout the body, zinc helps the immune system fight off invading bacteria and viruses. The body also needs zinc to make proteins and DNA, the genetic material in all cells. A serving of acai pulp provides 0.22 mg.

ROLE IN SUPPORTING HEALTH

KILLS CANCER CELLS: A study on leukemia cells conducted at University of Florida, Gainesville, and published in the January 2006 issue of *Journal of Agricultural and Food Chemistry*, showed that extracts from acai berries triggered a self-destruct response in up to 86 percent of leukemia cells tested. Researchers attributed the actions to acai's strong antioxidant makeup, due in large part to high concentrations of anthocyanins, a type of nutritious phytochemical that also gives acai berries their deep purple color.

SCAVENGES FREE RADICALS: Acai berries contain a large concentration of vitamins and phytochemicals called antioxidants. These phytochemicals help neutralize cell-damaging free radicals that create inflammation in the body, weaken the immune system, and over time, cause various signs of aging. Researchers at the Department of Nutrition and Food Science at Texas A&M University showed that acai berries possess the highest antioxidant activity of any fruit known to date, which allow the body to neutralize free radicals that can lead to degenerative diseases such as macular degeneration and Alzheimer's disease. The study was published in the June 2008 issue of the *Journal of Agricultural and Food Chemistry*.

STRENGTHENS THE IMMUNE SYSTEM: After studying the disease-preventing power of acai berries, scientists at the Department of Immunology and Infectious Diseases at Montana State University isolated a polysaccharide called arabinogalactan that is known to induce T cell activity. In lay terms, T cells are a type of white blood cell produced in the thymus. When made active by various unhealthy components or actions, T cells begin destroying healthy cells, which in turn weakens the immune system, leaving it vulnerable to infection. The study was published in the March 2012 issue of the peer-review journal *PLOS Pathogens*.

REDUCES CHOLESTEROL AND BLOOD SUGAR: In a study published in the May 2011 issue of *Nutrition Journal*, researchers from Medicus Research, Northridge, California, and UCLA School of Medicine, Department of Medicine, Los Angeles, California, gave ten overweight adults two 100-g servings of acai pulp daily for one month. While participants did not lose significant weight, they did reduce their fasting levels of plasma glucose, insulin, and total cholesterol, leaving researchers encouraged by the use of acai to regulate these health conditions.

SUPPLIES A GENEROUS SOURCE OF MINERALS: A 2014 article in the *Journal of Toxicology and Environmental Health* explored the amount of essential minerals found in acai pulp made from the berries gathered from various locations. The researchers' findings? Acai berries are rich in magnesium, zinc, calcium, and iron, as well as surprisingly high levels of manganese and copper (for a fruit).

GENERAL INFORMATION ABOUT ACAI

Acai berries are highly perishable and very fragile, which means the only way to eat them fresh is to actually visit the Amazon and eat them there. To enjoy the health benefits of acai berries, use the pulp—usually sold frozen—dried berries, acai juice, or acai berry powder.

STORAGE: If you have an opportunity to eat fresh berries, enjoy them on the spot. They begin to break down a day after being picked.

USAGE: Acai juice and pulp—typically sold frozen—are fantastic in smoothies or blended into sorbets and slushies. The dried berries are fun to toss into muffin, pancake, and waffle batter or into a pot of cooking quinoa, rice, or millet.

BOTANICAL BACKGROUND: Known scientifically as *Euterpe oleracea Martius*, acai is a member of the Arecaceae family (also known as the Palmae family). Acai berries grow on the same palm tree that provides hearts of palm.

GROWING INFORMATION: Acai berries grow in the wet soil of the Amazon basin on a slender 3-foot (1 m) tall palm tree. The tree matures at two or three years and begins producing a year-round supply of fruit, with the heaviest production in June and November, the two harvest periods.

HISTORY: For centuries, natives of the Amazon have eaten acai as a staple food. The berry's popularity broadened when Brazilian food scientists discovered, in the early 1980s, that acai berries retain their nutrition when frozen. With that information, frozen berry puree began showing up in Rio de Janeiro and other Brazilian cities, where it was touted as a natural energy booster. In 2008, there were more than fifty-three acai-containing products on the market in the United States and sales of foods containing acai surpassed $106 million.

THINGS TO BE AWARE OF: If you're scheduled to have a magnetic resonance imaging (MRI) test, it's important to let your doctor know if you've been eating acai berries, as very large doses of acai might affect the results of MRI scans.

STEPHANIE'S FAVORITE USES: I often use a teaspoon or two of dehydrated acai powder to make purple frosting for my kids' birthday cupcakes. I also like to add dried berries to trail mix and homemade granola.

ACAI: DID YOU KNOW?

- Acai berries grow on the same type of palm tree that is cultivated for hearts of palm.
- Acai berries are the most financially important non-wood crop in the Amazon.
- The leaves of the acai palm are used commercially. They are made into hats, mats, baskets, brooms, and roof thatch for homes.
- Because the wood of the acai palm resists pests, it is prized in building construction.
- Oil from acai berry seeds is used in shampoos, soaps, and skin moisturizers.

BLACKBERRIES

NUTRITION PROFILE

PER SERVING: (145 g)

BACKGROUND: Blackberries are some of the most antioxidant-dense berries around. This soft, sweet berry grows wild throughout North America and is a favorite wild-sourced food. Generations of Americans and Canadians grew up picking blackberries with their friends and families. In a pinch, blackberries can be used in place of raspberries. (The color of the finished dish won't look the same, but it will taste just as delicious.)

CALORIES: 43

FIBER: With 7 g of fiber, one serving of blackberries can help you reduce the risk of colon cancer and diverticular disease as well as help you feel satiated so you don't overeat.

PROTEIN: A serving of blackberries provides 2 g of protein, which helps to build and repair tissue.

VITAMIN A: A serving of blackberries provides 308 IUs of vitamin A, a nutrient that plays a vital role in bone growth, reproduction, and immune system health.

VITAMIN C: A 2007 study published in the *American Journal of Clinical Nutrition* found that middle-aged women who consumed vitamin C from food sources appeared

NUTRIENTS: HOW MUCH DO YOU NEED?

Name a nutrient—any nutrient—and chances are good that, depending on your age and gender, you will need different amounts of it. That is why the USDA created nutritional guidelines, for most nutrients, in the form of RDA or adequate intake (AI). Here is a list of nutrients found in berries, along with the USDA's AI suggestions.

Note: The USDA breaks down RDAs into very narrow groups and also offers suggestions for larger, more general groups, as shown here.

	MEN OVER THE AGE OF 18	WOMEN OVER THE AGE OF 18	PREGNANT WOMEN
FIBER	38 g	25 g	28 g
PROTEIN	56 g	26 g	71 g
VITAMIN A	900 IUs	700 IUs	770 IUs
VITAMIN B_6	1.3 mg	1.3 mg	1.9 mg
VITAMIN C	90 mg	75 mg	85 mg
VITAMIN E	15 mg	15 mg	15 mg
VITAMIN K	120 g	90 g	90 g
FOLATE	400 g	400 g	600 g
THIAMINE	1.2 mg	1.1 mg	1.4 mg
RIBOFLAVIN	1.3 mg	1.1 mg	1.4 mg
NIACIN	16 mg	15 mg	16 mg
CALCIUM	1,000 mg	1,000 mg	1,000 mg
IRON	18 mg	18 mg	27 mg
MAGNESIUM	400 mg	310 mg	350 mg
PHOSPHORUS	700 mg	700 mg	700 mg
POTASSIUM	4.7 g	4.7 g	4.7 g
ZINC	11 mg	8 mg	11 mg
SELENIUM	55 mcg	55 mcg	60 mcg

to have younger-looking skin with fewer wrinkles and less dryness than women who did not consume vitamin C-rich foods. A serving of blackberries will give you 30.2 mg of vitamin C.

VITAMIN E: This important antioxidant vitamin improves immune system function, helps lower your risk of cancer, and reduces blood cholesterol levels. You'll get 1.68 mg of vitamin E from a serving of blackberries.

VITAMIN K: This vitamin helps prevent and lessen the severity of osteoporosis, dementia, tooth decay, and infectious diseases such as pneumonia. A serving of blackberries provides 28.5 mcg of vitamin K.

FOLATE: A serving of blackberries provides 36 g of this B_9 vitamin, which is needed for the formation of red and white blood cells in bone marrow, the conversion of carbohydrates into energy, and the production of DNA and RNA.

CHOLINE: This micronutrient helps the body with nerve signaling, maintenance of cell membranes, and transporting triglycerides from the liver. A serving of blackberries provides 12.2 mg of choline.

COPPER: This mineral helps with the formation of collagen, increases the absorption of iron, and plays a role in energy production. A serving of blackberries provides 0.2 mg of copper.

MANGANESE: This mineral is involved in processing cholesterol, carbohydrates, and protein in the body. A serving of blackberries offers 0.9 mg of manganese.

ROLE IN SUPPORTING HEALTH

SUPPORTS OVERALL HEALTH: In a 2006 study published in the *American Journal of Clinical Nutrition*, scientists indicated that blackberries' antioxidant content of 5.75 millimoles (a clinical measurement indicating the amount of electrons and hydrogen atoms in a food) per serving was far above that of other foods. This means that regular consumption of blackberries may have a positive impact on overall health, athletic performance, and risk of disease.

MAY KILL CANCER CELLS: A team of researchers from Center for Human Nutrition, UCLA, Los Angeles, California, studied the effect of phytochemicals in berries on cancer cells. Blueberries, raspberries, cranberries, strawberries, and blackberries were studied. The berry with the strongest potential for cancer cell–killing ability? Blackberries. Results were published in the June 2006 issue of *Journal of Agricultural and Food Chemistry.*

IMPROVES BRAIN FUNCTION: In an animal study conducted by scientists from the USDA, blackberries appeared to spur improvements, not only in short-term memory but also in motor skills such as balance and coordination, which often decline with age. Researchers believe the polyphenols in blackberries may reduce inflammation and oxidation within aging neurons, which in turn makes it easier for brain cells to communicate with each other. The study was published in the January 2012 issue of *Journal of Agricultural and Food Chemistry.*

HELPS PREVENT COLON AND ESOPHAGEAL CANCERS: In a study published in the volume 60 2008 issue of *Nutrition and Cancer,* researchers at Ohio State University completed a study that showed a 60 to 80 percent reduction in colon tumors in rats fed a diet that included blackberries. Studies at Ohio State University showed an 80 percent reduction in esophageal cancers in mice fed a diet that included 5 to 10 percent blackberries. Scientists from Ohio State University are now conducting clinical trials into the effects of black raspberries on colon and esophageal cancer in humans.

IMPROVES ORAL HEALTH: Researchers at University of Kentucky College of Dentistry researched the antimicrobial effects of blackberries to see if they had any effect on oral herpes simplex virus. They significantly reduced oral lesions while preventing further outbreaks. This, and several similar studies on using blackberries to improve oral health, was published in the September 2011 issue of *Oral Surgery, Oral Medicine, Oral Pathology, Oral Radiology* magazine.

GENERAL INFORMATION ABOUT BLACKBERRIES

Blackberries are available fresh and frozen. Because berries stop ripening the moment they are picked, opt for already-ripe, brightly colored fruit that show no signs of weepiness, mold, or moisture. If you're purchasing frozen berries, go for unsweetened whole berries.

STORAGE: Do not wash blackberries until the moment you want to use them! Blackberries are highly perishable and should be stored (unwashed) for no more than two days before use. To store, remove any weepy, smashed, or moldy berries and put the unblemished fruit in a dry, shallow container. Lay a paper towel or clean dishtowel over the fruit and put the cover on securely. Place the container in the produce drawer or on a low shelf of your refrigerator. If you cannot use the berries within a couple days, place the container in the freezer for up to six months.

USAGE: When you are ready to use your berries, gently wash them with cool water. It's important to be gentle so you don't break the berries. Some people place berries in a colander, submerge it into a container or sink filled with cold water, and then allow the berries to drip dry. You can also mist the blackberries with a gentle stream of water. Pat them dry, if necessary, and use the berries immediately after washing them.

BOTANICAL BACKGROUND: Blackberries are vigorously growing members of the rose family. There are about forty species of blackberries, both wild and cultivated (beginning in the nineteenth century). They are grown throughout North America, Great Britain, Denmark, and Sweden. Unfortunately, identifying the different blackberry species is difficult because so many types of blackberry plants have crossbred by themselves. Many of the more recent varieties have been developed without the thorns that have made blackberry picking such a challenging activity.

HISTORY: Blackberries have been around for millennia, growing wild for most of history. The leaves and roots have been used as medicine, and the fruit has also been used for medicinal purposes—most commonly to treat constipation and help heal psoriasis and eczema. In 1696, the *London Pharmacopoeia* documented the use of blackberries to make wine and cordials.

GROWING INFORMATION: Blackberries grow on thorny, woody stems known as canes that grow into a tangle of brambles. Blackberries prefer fertile soil and a bit of coolness during the fall, winter, and spring.

THINGS TO BE AWARE OF: There are several berry varieties that claim to be related to the blackberry. One of these is the boysenberry (the berry I grew up on!), along with marionberries, olallieberries, and loganberries. Any of these berries can be used in recipes that call for blackberries in this book.

STEPHANIE'S FAVORITE USES: Blackberries are one of my favorites. I love them with a squirt of lime. I also love them in a few not-so-healthy ways, including tossed into a blended margarita (though I'll settle for sparkling water), tucked into an *aebleskiver* (a Danish sweet that is a cross between a donut hole and a pancake), and smooshed into coconut-milk ice cream.

BLUEBERRIES

NUTRITION PROFILE

PER SERVING: (150 g)

BACKGROUND: Blueberries are the second most popular berry in the United States after strawberries. A darling of the health-food crowd, the blueberry has garnered a lot of media attention over the last decade for its high levels of phytonutrients. Healthy food aficionados in the United Kingdom feel the same way: The blueberry, once an exotic North American rarity, has pushed raspberries out of the way to become Great Britain's second-favorite fruit, and British growers are raising more blueberries than ever before, with commercial production up 482 percent between 2008 and 2015.

CALORIES: 84

FIBER: A high-fiber diet can help reduce the risk of heart disease and diabetes, and maintain a healthy weight. A serving of blueberries provides 3.55 g of fiber.

VITAMIN C: Vitamin C helps protect cells and is involved in the production of collagen, which maintains healthy connective tissues and is important for the support and structure of tissues and organs, including the skin, bones, and blood vessels. A serving of blueberries will give you 14.36 mg of this important nutrient.

VITAMIN K: Known best for its role in healthy blood clotting, this vitamin also helps halt age-related bone loss. A serving of blueberries offers 28.56 mcg of vitamin K.

COPPER: One of the important functions of copper is to help in the production of red and white blood cells. A serving of blueberries gives you 0.08 mg of copper.

MANGANESE: Our bodies need a small amount of manganese each day to help form skin and bone cells and regulate blood sugar. A serving of blueberries will give you 0.5 mg of manganese.

ROLE IN SUPPORTING HEALTH

TREATS UTIs: Researchers at Rutgers University in New Jersey have identified a compound in blueberries that promotes urinary tract health and reduces the risk of infection. It appears to work by preventing bacteria from adhering to the cells that line the walls of the urinary tract. The study was published in the October 8, 1998, issue of the *New England Journal of Medicine*.

IMPROVES EYESIGHT: A number of studies in Europe have documented the relationship between bilberries, the European cousin of blueberries, and improved eyesight. This is thought to occur because of the anthocyanin in the blue pigment, which is also available in the blueberry. In Japan, blueberry supplements are common "eye strengthening" supplements, marketed to individuals who suffer from eye fatigue.

MAINTAINS YOUTH: Researchers at the USDA Human Nutrition Center (HNRCA), Beltsville, Maryland, have found that blueberries rank number one in antioxidant activity when compared to forty other fresh fruits and vegetables. Antioxidants help neutralize harmful by-products of metabolism called "free radicals" that can lead to cancer and other age-related diseases. In another HNRCA lab, neuroscientists discovered that feeding blueberries to laboratory rats slowed age-related loss in their mental capacity, a finding that has important implications for us. This research was published in the *USDA Database for the Oxygen Radical Absorbance Capacity (ORAC) of Selected Food* at www.ars.usda.gov/nutrientdata.

LOWERS BAD CHOLESTEROL: Blueberries reduce the buildup of so-called "bad" cholesterol that contributes to cardiovascular disease and stroke, according to a research study published in the October 1998 issue of *American Chemical Society* that was conducted at the University of California, Davis. Antioxidants are believed to be the active component.

GENERAL INFORMATION ABOUT BLUEBERRIES

When buying fresh blueberries, look for round, deeply colored fruit with a white bloom. Berries should be firm with no withered, soft, or weepy spots.

STORAGE: Like other berries, fresh blueberries should be kept in the refrigerator unwashed and completely dry until you are ready to use them. Pick out any blemished fruit and place the remaining berries in a shallow, covered container in the produce drawer of your refrigerator, where they will keep for about two days. For longer storage, place the container in the freezer, where you can keep the berries up to nine months.

USAGE: Blueberries can be washed immediately before use.

BOTANICAL BACKGROUND: Blueberries—members of the Ericaceae family—are related to cranberries and lingonberries. A small wild blueberry, called a bilberry, grows in Europe. Blueberries are native to North America.

HISTORY: North American blueberry bushes were exported to Europe for commercial cultivation in the 1930s.

GROWING INFORMATION: Blueberries grow on shrubs that can be as short as 4 inches (10 cm) for lowbush berries and

13 feet (4 m) for highbush berries. Like many berries, blueberries grow best in cool temperatures. The plants bear fruit usually between May and August.

THINGS TO BE AWARE OF: All the recipes in this book that call for blueberries can be made with wild blueberries or bilberries.

STEPHANIE'S FAVORITE USES: Because blueberries are so hardy, I love tossing a handful of frozen berries into a pot of cooking millet or quinoa or oats—they don't break and stain the grain like other berries do. Though a bit difficult to find, I love freeze-dried and dried blueberries. They are great in granola and trail mixes.

CRANBERRIES

NUTRITION PROFILE

PER SERVING: (100 g)

BACKGROUND: Cranberries were originally called crane berries, because early European settlers in North America believed this indigenous berry resembled the long-necked bird. These same settlers learned how to enjoy the berry from America's native people, who typically dried it and added it to other foods, such as dried meat. It was quickly discovered that if massive amounts of sweetener (such as honey or maple syrup) were added to these tart berries, they made a lovely dessert food. Dried cranberries and cranberry juice are popular ways to enjoy this healthy fruit, but do yourself a favor and avoid sweetened cranberries and sweetened cranberry juice (à la cranberry juice cocktail). Neither is a healthy food.

CALORIES: 46

FIBER: This important nutrient helps support digestive health and supports the good bacteria in your intestine, which in turn help your immune system work efficiently. A cup (100 g) of cranberries will provide 4.6 g of fiber.

VITAMIN C: This antioxidant vitamin supports your health in so many ways, including strengthening the immune system, keeping the cardiovascular system strong, and promoting healthy skin and gums. One cup (100 g) of cranberries provides 13.3 mg of vitamin C.

VITAMIN E: You'll get 1.2 mg from a serving of cranberries, which will help protect your body's cells from free radical damage as well as keep skin moist, supple, and healthy.

WHAT ARE PHYTONUTRIENTS?

Berries contain a lot of macronutrients (such as fiber) and even more micronutrients (vitamins, minerals, enzymes, amino acids, etc.). These important nutrients help keep us alive and have been heavily studied for decades. Not only do we know what they are, but also we know what they do and how much of each we need to be our healthiest. However, there is another type of nutrient that isn't as well known: Phytonutrients, or phytochemicals (*phyto* from the Greek word for *plant*), are the ingredients that give plants their colors, flavors, and fragrances. These substances also help protect plants from germs, fungi, bugs, and other threats. And while phytonutrients aren't essential to keeping humans alive, they are so powerful that they help prevent and reverse disease as well as slow aging and keep our bodies working properly. Because they haven't been studied for as long as fiber, protein, vitamins, and minerals, scientists haven't named—or even isolated—some of them. (At this writing, scientists believe there are more than 25,000 phytonutrients.)

We're learning more and more about phytonutrients daily, but for now, I can tell you this: Phytonutrients are powerful antioxidants and anti-inflammatory ingredients, and berries are one of the densest sources of these beneficial substances. Some of the phytonutrients in berries include these single phytochemicals and phytochemical families: ellagic acid, resveratrol, anthocyanins (which give berries their blue and red color), phenolic acids, proanthocyanidins, flavonoids, triterpenoids, carotenoids, glucosinolates, and phytoestrogens.

VITAMIN K: This fat-soluble vitamin is essential, ensuring that your blood clots properly when you bruise or cut yourself. A serving of cranberries provides 5.1 mcg of vitamin K.

COPPER: This essential trace mineral helps with the formation of collagen, increases the absorption of iron, and plays a role in energy production. A serving of cranberries provides 0.06 mg of copper.

MANGANESE: A serving of cranberries provides 0.36 mg of manganese, a mineral that supports healthy bone structure and bone metabolism and also helps create essential enzymes for building bones.

PANTOTHENIC ACID: Also known as vitamin B_5, pantothenic acid helps prevent and treat a number of health conditions, including asthma, hair loss, allergies, stress and anxiety, respiratory disorders, and heart problems. You'll get 0.29 mg of pantothenic acid from one serving of cranberries.

ROLE IN SUPPORTING HEALTH

HELPS FIGHT DIET-INDUCED OBESITY, INSULIN RESISTANCE, AND INTESTINAL INFLAMMATION: In September 2015, scientists from a number of Canadian medical schools and hospitals—including the Department of Medicine, Cardiology Axis of the Quebec Heart and Lung Institute and the Institute of Nutrition and Functional Foods, Laval University, both in Quebec, Canada—conducted an eight-week study on mice. One group of mice was fed a high-fat, high-sucrose diet, which is associated with a number of health conditions in humans, from obesity to diabetes. Half of the mice also received a daily dose of cranberry extract, while the other half did not. The mice that received the cranberry extract showed reduced weight gain compared to the control group. Daily treatment with cranberry extract also lowered triglyceride levels, improved insulin tolerance, and reduced inflammation in the intestinal tract. This study was published in the June 2015 issue of the gastroenterology journal *Gut*.

WARDS OFF UTIs: There have been dozens of studies on cranberry products and UTIs. Most have shown that cranberry juice does indeed shorten and lessen symptoms of an established UTI. A study published in the January 2014 issue of *Clinical Infectious Diseases* proved that cranberries can also prevent a UTI from occurring. For one year, researchers from UCLA followed 150 sexually active women, ages twenty-one to seventy-two, who had experienced three or more UTIs per year. One-third of the women received cranberry juice daily, another third received cranberry extract tablets every day, and a third group of women received a placebo. The groups that were give daily doses of cranberry juice or cranberry extract tablets showed a decrease in infections, symptoms, and antibiotic use; 20 percent of the juice group and 18 percent of the cranberry extract tablet group experienced a UTI; 32 percent of the placebo group experienced one or more infections during the study period.

LESSENS SYMPTOMS OF INFLAMMATORY BOWEL DISORDER (IBD): A group of researchers from Yale University, University of Massachusetts, and University of Korea studied the ability of various foods to lessen symptoms of inflammatory bowel disease in rats. They found that cranberry extract tablets and dried unsweetened cranberries significantly lessened IBD symptoms. The study also showed that dried cranberries were slightly more effective than cranberry extract tablets. This study was published in the January 2015 issue of *Food Chemistry*.

TREATS STREP THROAT: Researchers from Sri Gobind Tricentenary Dental College and Research Institute, Haryana, India, created a mouthwash containing cranberry extracts. They gave cranberry mouthwash to a group of twenty children, who had strep bacteria in their throats and mouths, and a placebo mouthwash to a control group of twenty children with strep bacteria in their throats and mouths. After four weeks of daily use, the group using cranberry mouthwash saw a significant decrease in the amount of strep throat symptoms and strep bacteria in the mouth and throat. This study was published in the 2015 volume 33 issue of *Journal of Indian Society of Pedodontics & Preventative Dentistry*.

HELPS LOWER BLOOD PRESSURE: Cranberries may even help lower blood pressure. A team of researchers from Agricultural Research Service, USDA, Beltsville, Maryland, conducted a double-blind study of thirty-six overweight women and twenty-five overweight men all in their fifties with body mass indexes of twenty-eight. Half of the individuals was given a placebo juice daily; the other half was given a low-calorie cranberry juice each day. At the end of eight weeks, the group that received cranberry juice showed lower blood pressure, lower triglycerides, and lower blood cholesterol levels than the control group. The results were published in the *Journal of Nutrition*, June 2014.

GENERAL INFORMATION ABOUT CRANBERRIES

When buying fresh berries, look for round, deeply colored fruit with no withered, soft, or weepy spots. One easy way to tell the freshness of a berry is to drop it. If it bounces, it's fresh and healthy. If it doesn't bounce, it is probably dehydrated and old or overly soft. When buying frozen cranberries or a bag of fresh berries, take a good look at the berries inside the bag. Most of them should be a bright red and unblemished.

STORAGE: Like other berries, fresh cranberries should be kept in the refrigerator unwashed and completely dry until you are ready to use them. Remove any blemished fruit and place the remaining berries in a shallow, covered container in the produce drawer of your refrigerator, where they will keep for about five to seven days. For longer storage, place the container in the freezer, where you can keep the cranberries up to nine months.

USAGE: Cranberries can be washed immediately before use. While most recipes that call for fresh or frozen cranberries suggest cooking them with a large amount of sweetener, more and more people are enjoying the tart charms of this berry when eaten raw.

BOTANICAL BACKGROUND: Cranberries are a member of the family Ericaceae, which also includes other berries, such as blueberries, bilberries, huckleberries, and lingonberries.

HISTORY: Cranberries have a long history as a food and medicine in North America, where they were used by Native Americans in various forms—fresh, juiced, boiled and mashed, and dried—both alone and mixed in with other foods, such as dried meat. They were also used in poultices to heal wounds and as a dye. The Algonquians called the berry *Sassamanash* and are said to be responsible for introducing cranberries to some of the first Europeans who settled in what is today Massachusetts. Soon, cranberries became a staple in the diet of the settlers and were mentioned in books and stories as well as recipe books. Barrels of cranberries—fresh and dried—were even sent back to England. Today, after many decades of playing a starring role at Thanksgiving and Christmas dinners, cranberries are now recognized as a superfood filled with phytonutrients that help support good health.

GROWING INFORMATION: Cranberries like moist soil and a cool climate, hence the concentration of commercial growers in eastern Canada, New England, some Mid-Atlantic states, and the Great Lakes region. Cranberries grow wild in bogs and other wetlands, but for commercial purposes they are now cultivated in constructed raised beds in areas that are surrounded by tables of water or irrigation ditches.

THINGS TO BE AWARE OF: Cranberries also contain a significant amount of salicylic acid, which is the same active ingredient found in aspirin. You should not drink a lot of cranberry juice if you are allergic to aspirin. If you take Warfarin, or other prescription medications, talk to your doctor before drinking cranberry juice. Mixing the juice with some medications can lessen the medication's effectiveness.

STEPHANIE'S FAVORITE USES: I love tart foods and enjoy making a Mexican-inspired relish for poultry with a roughly chopped handful of cranberries and walnuts, some red onion, cilantro, and a bit of apple cider vinegar. I also toss in a handful of chopped cranberries when making apple crisps or pies, and anytime I want to kill a chocolate craving I do so by tossing a handful of cranberries into my juicer with one or two whole lemons and a handful of baby salad greens.

CRANBERRIES: THE HOLIDAY BERRY

Americans consume about 80 million pounds of cranberries during Thanksgiving week, and 94 percent of their Thanksgiving dinners include cranberry sauce.

CURRANTS, BLACK

NUTRITION PROFILE

PER SERVING: fresh (110 g)

BACKGROUND: A relative of the gooseberry, black currants are glossy, black, round fruit, and are best used fresh. If you're at the store, or shopping online, and see frozen black currants or canned or jarred black currants that have been cooked in sugar syrup or corn syrup, avoid them. They are too high in sugar to be healthy.

Note: Dried currants, sometimes called Zante currants, are actually petite, dried grapes, not currants.

CALORIES: 71

PROTEIN: Without adequate protein, our bodies can't put together the structures that make up cells, tissue, and organs. A serving of black currants will provide 2 g of protein.

OMEGA-3 FATTY ACIDS: A serving of black currants provides 80.6 mg of omega-3 fatty acids, which regulate the function of the cell receptors in membranes throughout the body.

VITAMIN C: This important vitamin helps the body form and maintain connective tissue between skin, ligaments, cartilage, bones, and teeth. A serving of black currants provides 203 mg of vitamin C.

IRON: This important mineral is necessary for growth, development, normal cellular functioning, and synthesis of some hormones and connective tissue. You'll get 1.7 mg of iron from a serving of black currants.

POTASSIUM: Black currants provide 361 mg of potassium per serving. This essential mineral is a major electrolyte. It plays an important role in electrolyte regulation, nerve function, muscle control, and blood pressure.

MANGANESE: A serving of black currants gives you 0.3 mg of manganese, a mineral that helps in collagen production. Collagen is the protein that makes up skin. Manganese also functions as an antioxidant in skin cells.

ROLE IN SUPPORTING HEALTH

KILLS CANCER CELLS: In a study on liver cells, researchers from Northeastern Ohio Universities Colleges of Medicine and Pharmacy, Rootstown, Ohio, studied the effect of black currant extract on cancerous liver cells. After being exposed to black currant extract in the laboratory, the cells stopped proliferating and died. Researchers suspect that the anthocyanins, a phytonutrient in black currants, are responsible. The study was published in the October 2012 issue of *Natural Product Communications* journal.

SUPPORTS RECOVERY AFTER EXERCISE: In a 2009 study published in the July 2009 issue of *American Journal of Physiology*, researchers from the New Zealand Institute for Plant and Food Research, Ltd., Hamilton, New Zealand, gave test subjects black currant capsules, equal to about ⅓ cup (35 g) berries, pre- and post-exercise, for three weeks and had them do a variety of exercises. The results showed significantly lower levels of biomarkers of oxidative stress in plasma and significantly increased ability of plasma to suppress inflammatory responses. Researchers found that black currants boost the natural benefits of exercise by reducing muscle damage and soreness and assist immune protection, allowing exercisers to train harder for longer periods. This is one of several studies linking black currants with faster exercise recovery time. Researchers from the University of Chichester, UK, asked fourteen male test subjects to cycle each day at a moderate pace for 16.1 km (10 miles). The group that received daily black currant extract improved their time trial performance and fat oxidation. This study was published in the *European Journal of Applied Physiology*, November 2015.

HELPS GLAUCOMA PATIENTS: Several studies have focused on the effect of black currants on glaucoma and eye health in general. In a trial that was published in the

November 2007 issue of *Hirosaki Medical Journal*, researchers from Hirosaki University Graduate School of Hirosaki, Japan, looked at the effect of black currant anthocyanins on blood flow in the retina of patients with normal-tension glaucoma. Glaucoma is usually associated with high intraocular eye pressure. After consuming 50 mg of black currant anthocyanins per day for six months, test subjects showed significantly increased blood flows at key sites in the eye and none showed an advancement of the disease.

SUPPORTS GUT HEALTH AND PREVENTION OF COLON CANCER: Black currants have long been a folk remedy for improved gut health. In a study published in the March 2014 issue of *Phytotherapy Research* and performed by scientists at Massey University, Palmerston North, New Zealand, the intestinal bacteria of thirty healthy men and women were analyzed. Test subjects were then given black currant extract. The result? A significant increase in the population of helpful intestinal bacteria and a decrease in the activity of toxic bacterial enzymes that are associated with colon cancer. The results also showed significantly decreased fecal pH (high fecal pH is thought to be a risk for colon cancer).

DECREASES VASCULAR INFLAMMATION: A 2008 study performed by researchers from University of Southern Denmark, in Odense, showed that black currant and orange juice decreased vascular inflammation and the risk of cardiovascular disorder. For twenty-eight days, researchers gave a black currant–orange juice mixture to individuals who suffered from peripheral arterial disease, a common circulatory problem in which narrowed blood vessels reduce blood flow to the arms and legs. At the end of the trial, test subjects saw an 11 percent decrease in C-reactive protein and a 3 percent decrease in fibrinogen, both indicators of inflammation in the veins. The study was published in the January 2009 issue of *British Journal of Nutrition*.

GENERAL INFORMATION ABOUT BLACK CURRANTS

When buying fresh black currants, look for round, deeply colored fruit with a nice gloss. Berries should be firm with no withered, soft, or weepy spots.

STORAGE: Fresh black currants should be kept in the refrigerator unwashed and completely dry until you are ready to use them. Remove any blemished fruit and place berries in a shallow, covered container in the produce drawer of your refrigerator, where they will keep for about two days. For longer storage, place the container in the freezer for up to nine months.

USAGE: Black currants can be washed immediately before being used.

BOTANICAL BACKGROUND: The black currant is a woody shrub in the Grossulariaceae family, which grows wild in temperate areas of northern and central Europe and Asia. It is cultivated in Great Britain, Europe, and North America.

HISTORY: Black currants have been eaten as food and used as medicine for millennia. Perhaps some of the most interesting black currant stories, however, date from World War II. In wartime Great Britain, oranges and other vitamin C-rich foods were nearly impossible to come by. However, the United Kingdom had ample supplies of black currants, which contain high levels of vitamin C and are well suited to the climate in England. The British government asked citizens to step things up by growing their own black currants. Soon the country had enough to keep soldiers and citizens healthy, despite other food shortages. In fact, from 1942 onward, black currant syrup was distributed free of charge to children under the age of two.

GROWING INFORMATION: It prefers damp fertile soils, temperate climates, and while cold hardy, a moderately warm spring. Harvest time is mid- to late summer.

STEPHANIE'S FAVORITE USES: I love black currants with pork, sweet potatoes, and winter squash. I also like to use them in sorbet.

CURRANTS, RED

NUTRITION PROFILE

PER SERVING: fresh (110 g)

BACKGROUND: Beautiful red currants have a bright, bracing flavor, thanks to their high acidity. Red, round, and glossy, red currants are prized for their vitamin C content as well as their flavor. In Europe, using red currants to dress up rich meats and poultry is a popular, long-standing tradition.

CALORIES: 63

PROTEIN: At 2 g of protein per serving, red currants have a moderate amount of protein, the macronutrient responsible for helping the body build and repair itself.

FIBER: A serving of red currants provides 5 g of fiber, a quantity that has been found to lower the risk of colorectal cancer and other gastrointestinal cancers.

OMEGA-3 FATTY ACIDS: This essential fatty acid plays an important role in brain function and may help fight against cardiovascular disease. A serving of red currants boasts 39.2 mg of omega-3 fatty acids.

VITAMIN C: Vitamin C improves the absorption of iron from plant-based foods and helps the immune system work properly to protect the body from disease. A serving of red currants provides 45.9 mg of vitamin C.

VITAMIN K: This vitamin assists the transport of calcium throughout the body. It may also help reduce bone loss and decrease risk of bone fractures. A serving of red currants offers 12.3 mcg of vitamin K.

POTASSIUM: A mineral crucial to body functions, it plays an important role in electrolyte regulation, nerve function, muscle control, and blood pressure. One cup of red currants provides 308 mg of potassium.

MANGANESE: This mineral helps the body form connective tissue, bones, blood clotting factors, and sex hormones. A serving of red currants will provide 0.2 mg of manganese.

ROLE IN SUPPORTING HEALTH

HELPS WITH WEIGHT LOSS AND KEEPS THE PANCREAS HEALTHY:

Pancreatic lipase is an enzyme that breaks down fat in the blood so that the body may be able to absorb and utilize that fat. However, several commercial dieting products claim to block pancreatic lipase. The thinking is: It may be easier to lose weight if the body doesn't absorb fats from food (and the calories that come with these fats). Researchers at Łódź University of Technology, Łódź, Poland, studied the effects of several foods on pancreatic lipase and found that red currant juice naturally inhibited the production of pancreatic lipase, leading researchers to consider using red currant as a natural weight-loss aid. This study was published in the September 2015 issue of *Plant Foods For Human Nutrition*.

PROTECTS AGAINST CANCER, HEART DISEASE, AND DIABETES:

Oxidative cell damage contributes to the development of atherosclerosis, cancer, diabetes, and many other diseases. Researchers from University of Kaiserslautern, Kaiserslautern, Germany, wanted to see if anthocyanins—the phytonutrients that give red currants (and other red and purple fruits) their bright color—could help prevent health conditions. Eighteen healthy men were recruited and asked to drink a special solution each day for three weeks. One half of the group received 3 cups (700 ml) of an anthocyanin-rich juice, while the other half of the group acted as the control group and received a placebo drink. DNA samples were analyzed. The results: Anthocyanin clearly reduced oxidative cell damage in healthy men, while the placebo juice did nothing to reduce oxidative cell damage in the control group. This study was published in the April 2006 issue of *Biotechnology Journal*.

GENERAL INFORMATION ABOUT RED CURRANTS

When buying fresh red currants, look for round, brightly colored fruit with a nice gloss. Berries should be firm with no withered, soft, or weepy spots.

STORAGE: Like other berries, fresh red currants should be kept in the refrigerator unwashed and completely dry until you are ready to use them. Remove any blemished fruit and place the remaining berries in a shallow, covered container in the produce drawer of your refrigerator, where they will keep for about two days. For longer storage, place the container in the freezer, where you can keep the berries up to nine months.

USAGE: Red currants can be washed immediately before being used.

BOTANICAL BACKGROUND: Red currants are related to black currants and gooseberries. A member of the Grossulariaceae family, the red currant is native to western and northern Europe and grows wild throughout Asia.

HISTORY: Though red currants grow wild on many continents, it's believed they were first cultivated in Scandinavia and introduced to England in the late sixteenth century. In 1639, the red berries traveled overseas to the Massachusetts Bay Colony. Not only did these tart treats make their way into sweets and sauces, but also they were used as medicine (a popular preventative remedy for scurvy) and clothing dye.

GROWING INFORMATION: Red currants like well-drained soil; cool, humid summers; and a cool winter. In fact, many farmers say a frost gives berries their sweetness.

THINGS TO BE AWARE OF: The white currant is an albino version of the red currant, not a separate species. A bit milder in taste than its red sibling and with slightly lower antioxidant levels, it still a healthy, delicious berry.

STEPHANIE'S FAVORITE USES: I love rødgrød, a sweet soup made with red currants and other red berries. Yum!

ELDERBERRIES

NUTRITION PROFILE

PER SERVING: (145 g)

BACKGROUND: Known in the healing world as Sambuca, elderberry is packed with a generous amount of phytonutrients. It is a favorite healing plant, boiled into a delicious syrup and enjoyed daily to strengthen the immune system, or taken as a natural cold and flu remedy.

CALORIES: 106

PROTEIN: This macronutrient is vital to the maintenance of body tissue, including development and repair. A serving of elderberries will give you 1 g of protein.

FIBER: A serving of elderberries provides 10.2 g of fiber, a nutrient that helps move food through the stomach and intestines and adds bulk to stools.

OMEGA-3 FATTY ACIDS: Also known as polyunsaturated fatty acids, these play a crucial role in brain function as well as normal growth and development. A serving of elderberries provides 123 mg of omega-3 fatty acids.

VITAMIN A: This vitamin is needed for new cell growth and healthy skin, hair, and tissues. A serving of elderberries gives you 870 IU of vitamin A.

VITAMIN B$_6$: Also known as pyridoxine, this nutrient converts food into glucose, which is used to produce energy and make neurotransmitters. These neurotransmitters in turn carry signals from one nerve cell to another. A serving of elderberries offers 0.3 mg of vitamin B$_6$.

VITAMIN C: A serving of elderberries gives you 52.2 g of this important vitamin, which makes collagen, an important protein in skin, cartilage, tendons, ligaments, and blood vessels.

IRON: This mineral helps the body store and transport oxygen to all of the tissues, and also protects cells against the damaging effects of free radicals. A serving of elderberries provides 2.3 mg of iron.

POTASSIUM: It helps the body to conduct electricity, which is crucial to heart function and muscle contraction. You will get 406 mg of this mineral from a serving of elderberries.

ROLE IN SUPPORTING HEALTH

HELPS TREAT DIABETES: Researchers from University of Ulster, Coleraine, in northern Ireland studied elderberry's ability to stabilize blood sugar in diabetic mice that were given an extract of the berry. The results demonstrated the presence of insulin-releasing and insulin-like activity in the elderberry, a plant that traditional healers have used to address diabetes. The study was published in the *Journal of Nutrition*, 2000.

WARDS OFF INFLUENZA: Walk down the "cold and flu" aisle of any pharmacy and you'll see elderberry products. Does the berry work to combat flus? Research says yes. In a Norwegian trial, sixty male and female patients between the ages of eighteen and fifty-four years old were recruited during the Norwegian flu season (between December and February) from four primary-care sites in Norway to study the efficacy of standardized elderberry syrup for the treatment of influenza. All volunteers selected for the study had a fevers and respiratory symptoms. Patients were randomized to receive either a standardized black elderberry syrup or a placebo syrup, of which they took 15 ml, four times a day. By days three and four of the trial, the elderberry group was reporting greatly diminished or nonexistent symptoms, while the placebo group didn't report reduced or nonexistent symptoms until days seven to ten. The study was published in the 2004 issue of the *Journal of International Medical Research.*

In an Israeli trial published in the 1995 issue of the *Journal of Alternative and Complementary Medicine,* researchers studied seventeen adults and children with flu symptoms. Half of the group received elderberry syrup (adults took four tablespoons a day and children under the age of twelve took two tablespoons a day), while the other half received a placebo. Within two days, 93.3 percent of the elderberry group experienced a significant improvement of symptoms, including reduction of fever, compared to 91.7 percent of the placebo group, which did not show improvement until day six. The complete disappearance of symptoms was achieved within two to three days in approximately 90 percent of the elderberry group and within six days in the placebo group.

MAKES WEIGHT LOSS EASIER: Elderberries might help get you into your skinny jeans, based on a study performed by C. Chrubasik in the Institute of Forensic Medicine at the University of Freiburg in Germany. The analysis included eighty individuals who had a daily dose of elderberry juice enriched with elderberry blossom and berry powder extracts. Test subjects not only lost fat, but also experienced lowered blood pressure as well. The study was published in the April 2015 issue of *Phytotherapy Research.*

TREATS FUNGAL INFECTIONS: In the May 2010 issue of *Molecules,* a team of researchers from Kyungpook National University, Daegu, Korea, investigated the fungus-fighting ability of a compound called pinoresinol, a phytonutrient isolated from elderberry. Researchers found that pinoresinol is a powerful fungus figher, even killing strong fungus such as Candida, a yeast that causes thrush when present in the mouth and yeast infections when present in the genital tract.

GENERAL INFORMATION ABOUT ELDERBERRIES

When buying fresh elderberries, look for round, deeply colored fruit with a nice gloss. Berries should be firm with no withered, soft, or weepy spots.

STORAGE: Like other berries, fresh elderberries should be kept in the refrigerator unwashed and completely dry until you are ready to use them. Remove any blemished fruit and place the remaining berries in a shallow, covered container in the produce drawer of your refrigerator, where they will keep for about two days. For longer storage, place the container in the freezer, where you can keep the berries up to nine months.

USAGE: Elderberries can be washed immediately before being used.

BOTANICAL BACKGROUND: The elderberry, or *Sambucus*, as it is known scientifically, is a flowering plant shrub in the Adoxaceae family.

HISTORY: Elderberries have a long and illustrious history in Europe and North America as a healing food.

GROWING INFORMATION: Elderberries typically grow wild, often near dwellings, and are sometimes planted as a barrier or hedge. As long as they receive enough light, elderberries happily grow in a variety of soils. Berries are harvested summer through autumn.

THINGS TO BE AWARE OF: The ripe, cooked berries (pulp and skin) of elderberries are edible. However, uncooked berries and other parts of the elderberry plant are poisonous. In 1984, a group of twenty-five people were made sick, apparently by elderberry juice pressed from fresh, uncooked berries, leaves, and stems.

STEPHANIE'S FAVORITE USES: I love elderberry syrup stirred into a glass of sparkling water (my kids like it on waffles). I also enjoy mixing equal parts elderberry syrup and water and freezing it into ice cubes that are great in sparkling drinks.

GOJI BERRIES

NUTRITION PROFILE

PER SERVING: dried (28 g)

BACKGROUND: Though goji juice and goji powder are both health-food staples, these sweet-sour russet-colored berries are most often available dried. (They are too fragile to be shipped fresh from their native China.) How do they taste? Well, imagine a raisin crossed with a dried unsweetened cranberry, and you get a bright taste and satisfying chew. Dried goji berries can be found in 8-ounce and 1-pound pouches in supermarkets and health-food stores.

CALORIES: 90 calories

PROTEIN: This macronutrient is an important building block of bones, muscles, cartilage, skin, and blood. A serving of dried goji berries provides 4 g of protein.

FIBER: A high-fiber diet protects against hemorrhoids and helps prevent the development of small pouches in your colon (also known as diverticular disease). You'll get 4 g of fiber in one serving of dried goji berries.

VITAMIN A: This antioxidant vitamin plays an important role in the normal formation and maintenance of the heart, lungs, kidneys, and other vital organs. You'll receive 2520 IUs of vitamin A with every serving.

VITAMIN C: Gogi berries can help in improving dilation of blood vessels in people suffering from angina pectoris, congestive heart failure, and high blood pressure. One serving of these dried berries provides 5.4 mg of vitamin C.

IRON: This mineral helps metabolize proteins and plays a role in the production of hemoglobin and red blood cells. One serving of dried goji berries offers 4.4 mg of iron.

RIBOFLAVIN: Known as vitamin B_2, riboflavin is found in every human tissue and is necessary for processing amino acids and fats as well as breaking down carbohydrates. One serving of dried goji berries offers 0.4 mg of riboflavin.

SELENIUM: You'll receive 17.8 mcg of selenium from one serving of dried goji berries. This nutrient is involved in the production of prostaglandins in the body, which regulate inflammation levels.

ROLE IN SUPPORTING HEALTH

IMPROVES OVERALL WELL-BEING: In a double-blind study published in the May 14, 2008, issue of the *Journal of Alternative and Complementary Medicine*, scientists gave 120 ml (½ cup) of goji berry juice to one group and 150 ml (⅔ cup) of a placebo liquid to another group for fifteen consecutive days. At the end of the study, neither the goji group nor the placebo group showed any difference in weight. But the subjects who received goji berry juice daily reported increased energy levels; improved athletic performance; better quality of sleep and ease of awakening; more ability to focus on activities; greater mental acuity; calmness; and feelings of health, contentment, and happiness, as well as significantly reduced fatigue and stress. Subjects who received a placebo reported no difference in these areas.

IMPROVES IMMUNE-SYSTEM FUNCTION: A study published in the January 2009 issue of *Nutrition Research* journal shows the effects of daily goji berry consumption on healthy adults aged fifty-five to seventy-two years old. Fifty individuals took part in the study: Half were given 120 ml (½ cup) of a placebo drink and half of the group was given 120 ml (½ cup) of a goji berry drink. At the end of thirty days, the goji berry group showed increased antioxidant markers and lower oxidative damage, leading researchers to speculate that daily goji berry consumption can increase immune-system functioning.

STRENGTHENS THE IMMUNE SYSTEM AS WE AGE: In a study performed by researchers at Xinjiang Agricultural University, Urumqili City, China, artificially aged mice were given goji berry extract for thirty days in order to study age-induced oxidative stress in different organs. The findings: The immune function of organs was restored to normal age-appropriate function. The study was published in the May 2007 issue of *Journal of Ethnopharmacology*.

KEEPS TESTICLES AND OTHER TISSUE HEALTHY: In the category of "what were they thinking?," researchers from Dicle Üniversitesi, Diyarbakır, Turkey, created a state of testicular torsion in the testicles of lab rats. The study, published in the February 2015 issue of *International Journal of Clinical and Experimental Medicine*, reported that the rats that were given goji berry extract experienced less ischemic reperfusion injury (damage caused when blood supply returns to tissue after it has been deprived of oxygen) than the rats that did not receive goji berry extract. In other words, testicular torsion was reduced by the antioxidant effect of goji berry extract.

IMPROVES MEN'S SEXUAL HEALTH: Exposure to high levels of Bisphenol-A (BPA) has been linked to reproductive-organ damage in boys and men. In a study published in the December 2013 issue of *Evidence-Based Complementary and Alternative Medicine*, researchers from Chi Institute of Traditional Chinese Veterinary Medicine, Agricultural University of Hebei, China, examined goji berry's reputation as a sexual healing aid. The scientists fed BPA-exposed mice with goji berry extracts for seven days. The animals, which had experienced atrophied reproductive organs from the BPA exposure, recovered their testicular weight to near-normal levels.

GENERAL INFORMATION ABOUT GOJI BERRIES

Dried goji berries are easily found in health-food stores. Look for brands that do not contain added sweetener of any kind.

STORAGE: Dried goji berries can be kept in a tightly sealed bag in a dry place for up to six months.

USAGE: If your goji berries are on the dry, hard side, you may need to hydrate them before using. To do this, place them in a cup, pour a small amount of warm water over the berries (just enough to barely cover them), and let them soften for about twenty minutes. Rinse the berries (save the nutrient-dense liquid to drink or add to a recipe) and pat them dry. The berries are now ready to use.

BOTANICAL BACKGROUND: Native to Asia, goji berries are the fruit of the *Lycium barbarum* plant, a species of boxthorn in the nightshade family, Solanaceae. The family also includes potatoes, tomatoes, eggplants, belladonna, chile peppers, and tobacco.

HISTORY: Goji berries have been used as a medicine and as food (most often in soups) in China for thousands of years. Traditional Chinese medicine practitioners continue to use the berry as a liver tonic to heal the kidneys as well as a means of healing a host of male sexual disorders from impotence to atrophied testicles. Women have traditionally used the berry as a "beauty tea," which is said to make the skin look clear and firm.

GROWING INFORMATION: Goji berries are woody perennial plants that grow from one to three meters (3.25 to 9.75 feet) tall. The berries mature between July and October.

THINGS TO BE AWARE OF: Goji berry has a slight blood-thinning property, which makes it helpful for some people. However, if you are currently taking a blood thinner, please speak with your health-care provider before making goji a regular part of your diet.

STEPHANIE'S FAVORITE USES: I enjoy using dried goji berries in oatmeal cookies, granola, and trail mix.

GOOSEBERRIES

NUTRITION PROFILE

PER SERVING: (150 g)

BACKGROUND: Tart, firm, green, and round, gooseberries once enjoyed "favorite berry" status throughout the United Kingdom and the States. Today, they are considered a specialty berry that you can purchase in gourmet supermarkets or from local farmers (they are a bit fragile to ship long distances).

CALORIES: 66

PROTEIN: A serving of gooseberries provides 1.6 g of protein, a macronutrient that is necessary for the structure, function, and regulation of the body's tissues and organs.

FIBER: One of the many benefits of fiber is that it acts as food for the bacterial culture that makes up the mucosal lining of your large intestine, which protects the gastrointestinal wall and prevents inflammatory diseases such as colitis and Crohn's disease. A serving of gooseberries will give you 6 g of this important nutrient.

VITAMIN A: This vitamin helps maintain healthy skin, teeth, bones, soft tissue, mucus membranes, and skin. It is also known as retinol because it produces the pigments in the retina of the eye. You'll get 435 IUs of vitamin A from a serving of gooseberries.

VITAMIN C: A serving of gooseberries gives you 41.6 mg of this vitamin, which your body needs to make skin, tendons, ligaments, and blood vessels as well as to heal wounds and form scar tissue.

MANGANESE: This mineral helps the body create connective tissue, bones, blood clotting factors, and sex hormones. A serving of gooseberries provides 0.02 mg.

ROLE IN SUPPORTING HEALTH

HELPS MANAGE HYPERTENSION AND DIABETES: In a study published in the April 2010 issue of *Journal of Food Biochemistry*, a multinational team of researchers from *Universidade de São Paulo*, Brazil, and University of Massachusetts, Amherst, examined the antioxidants in gooseberries. Their findings: Based on their free radical scavenging ability, the major phenolic compounds of quercetin (in green gooseberries) and chlorogenic acid (in the less common red gooseberries) boasted potential antidiabetes and antihypertension functionality, making them an important treatment addition for individuals managing early stages of type 2 diabetes.

IMPROVES BRAIN HEALTH AND FUNCTION: A 2011 study by researchers from University of Seville, Spain, found that kaempferol—an antioxidant phytonutrient plentiful in gooseberries—has the ability to encourage brain cell growth. For the greatest benefit, enjoy gooseberries two or more times each week. This review was published in the April 2011 issue of *Mini-Reviews in Medicinal Chemistry*.

HELPS PREVENT CANCER: A study published in the February 2014 issue of *Food & Function* found that the quercetin and catechins in gooseberry help stop the growth of breast and colon cancer cells.

REDUCES INFLAMMATION: A team of researchers from Pusan National University, Busan, Republic of Korea, studied the effect of kaempferol, a phytonutrient found in gooseberries, on kidney tissue in aging rats. The study, published in a 2009 issue of *Journal of Medicinal Food*, involved feeding elderly rats kaempferol at 2 or 4 mg per kg of body weight daily for ten days. At the end of the study, it was shown that both amounts reduced inflammation in kidney tissue.

GENERAL INFORMATION ABOUT GOOSEBERRIES

When buying fresh berries, look for round, shiny fruit with no withered, soft, or weepy spots. Sometimes gooseberries are sold with their husks.

STORAGE: Fresh gooseberries should be kept in the refrigerator unwashed (and unhusked) until you are ready to use them. Remove any blemished fruit and place the berries in a shallow, covered container in the produce drawer of your refrigerator, where they will keep for about five to seven days. For longer storage, remove the fruit's husks and place the container in the freezer, where you can keep the berries up to nine months.

USAGE: Many gooseberries will come with husks, which you'll need to remove. After removing the husks, wash the berries thoroughly in cold water before cutting off the ends with a pair of kitchen scissors. Although most recipes that call for gooseberries suggest cooking them with large amounts of sweetener, try eating them raw—you might enjoy their tart charm.

BOTANICAL BACKGROUND: The gooseberry, known scientifically as *Ribes uva-crispa*, is related to red and black currants, which are also members of the *Ribes* genus.

HISTORY: Wild gooseberries have enjoyed a long history as a medicinal food, most commonly used to treat colds, excess sweating, scurvy, and stomach pain. Enjoyed since ancient times, gooseberries were not cultivated until the sixteenth century, when they became a favorite with British cooks and used for a variety of savory dishes and desserts. While they have since fallen out of favor—bumped out of first place by raspberries, blueberries, and strawberries— they still have an enthusiastic fan base!

GROWING INFORMATION: Gooseberries grow on 5-feet (1.5 meters) tall, thorny bushes in cool climates that have moderate summers. This hardy plant grows happily with little care but is also planted in cultivated rows.

THINGS TO BE AWARE OF: While gooseberries and currants are related, they are not interchangeable in recipes.

STEPHANIE'S FAVORITE USES: I like to combine a handful of gooseberries with blueberries when making pie, and I love cooking gooseberries in a bit of apple cider, until they're just soft, and then fold the compote into a cup or two of Whipped Coconut Cream (see page 150) to make an easy Gooseberry Fool.

LINGONBERRIES

NUTRITION PROFILE

PER SERVING: fresh (145 g)

BACKGROUND: These tart, glossy, red berries are a popular, wild-growing fruit in Scandinavia and other areas of northern Europe. Because they are sour, they are usually eaten cooked and sweetened or raw and mashed with sugar. They are available fresh from specialty markets and farmers' markets, or you can purchase them frozen.

CALORIES: 71

PROTEIN: Your body uses protein to build and repair tissues as well as to make enzymes, hormones, and other body chemicals. One serving of lingonberries provides 3 g of protein.

FIBER: Fiber helps food pass through the digestive system and adds bulk to the stool, which helps prevent constipation. A serving of lingonberries provides 3.7 g of fiber.

VITAMIN A: One serving of lingonberries provides 90 IUs of vitamin A, a nutrient that helps the heart, lungs, kidneys, and other organs work properly.

HAWTHORN BERRIES

Hawthorn berries are not particularly delicious and are rarely used for culinary purposes, but they do have a long history as a medicinal plant. The berries—and even the leaves and flowers—are brewed into a tea that is used to treat heart failure, chest pain, irregular heartbeat, high blood pressure, and hardening of the arteries. Indeed, a study published in the February 2002 issue of *Phytotherapy Research* found that hawthorn berry extract demonstrated measurable lowered blood pressure in individuals with mild high blood pressure. The magic ingredient in hawthorn berries? Heart-protective antioxidants, including quercetin and oligomeric procyandins. And while the hawthorn berry is considered safe, it can interfere with heart medication, so please speak to your health-care advisor before using it.

VITAMIN C: This powerful antioxidant helps the body form and maintain connective tissue, including bones, blood vessels, and skin. You'll get 64.8 mg of vitamin C from one serving of lingonberries.

ROLE IN SUPPORTING HEALTH

HELPS FIGHT CANCER: In a study published in the October 2001 issue of the *European Journal of Clinical Nutrition*, researchers from the National Public Health Institute in Helsinki, Finland, studied the effects of lingonberries and other dark berries on forty healthy men, aged sixty. Twenty of the subjects consumed 100 g/day of berries (lingonberries with black currants and bilberries) for eight weeks while the other twenty subjects continued eating their usual diet (which did not contain berries). Fasting blood samples were obtained from all the participants. In the trial group, serum (blood) concentration of quercetin was 32 to 51 percent higher compared with the control group. Quercetin, a phytonutrient found in lingonberries and other berries, is a powerful antioxidant that has been used, traditionally, to treat cancer.

HEALS DAMAGED BLOOD VESSELS: For eight weeks, researchers from University of Helsinki, Finland, gave rats with damaged blood vessels and high blood pressure lingonberry juice. At the end of the study, the rats' blood pressure had not changed, but the lining of their damaged blood vessels had healed. The study was published in the October 2011 issue of the *Journal of Functional Foods*.

LOWERS BLOOD SUGAR LEVELS: In a study performed by researchers at Université de Montréal, Quebec, Canada, diabetic members of the Cree people were given lingonberry extract—lingonberry being a traditional treatment for diabetes. The lingonberry extract reduced the by-product of sugars and protein by-products in the patients' blood that contribute to blood vessel damage, kidney disease, eye disease, circulation problems, sores, and amputation.

The study was published in the May 2010 issue of *Phytotherapy Research*.

RROTECTS AGAINST OXIDATIVE STRESS: Free radical damage ages our cells and tissues, making us look and feel older than we are and also making us more susceptible to infections and other disease. In a study published in the April 2011 issue of *Journal of Agricultural and Food Chemistry*, researchers from CHR-Hansen-SAS, Prades-le-Lez, France, fed rats a diet inducing oxidative stress. Supplementation with lingonberry extract significantly decreased oxidation in the body while increasing antioxidant defense enzymes in the blood and liver, confirming lingonberry's strong antioxidant activity.

GENERAL INFORMATION ABOUT LINGONBERRIES

When buying fresh lingonberries, look for round, brightly colored fruit. Berries should be firm with no withered, soft, or weepy spots. For your health's sake, avoid canned or jarred lingonberries cooked in syrup. If you can't find them fresh, buy frozen lingonberries and substitute them for the fresh product.

STORAGE: Like other berries, fresh lingonberries should be kept in the refrigerator unwashed and completely dry until you are ready to use them. Remove any blemished fruit and place the berries in a shallow, covered container in the produce drawer of your refrigerator, where they will keep for between one and two weeks. For longer storage, place the container in the freezer, where you can keep the berries up to nine months.

USAGE: Lingonberries can be washed immediately before being used.

BOTANICAL BACKGROUND: Members of the Ericaceae family, lingonberries are relatives of cranberries, blueberries, huckleberries, and bilberries. The name *lingonberry* originates from the Swedish name *lingon* for the species, and is derived from the Norse *lyngr*, or heather.

HISTORY: Lingonberries grow wild in northern Russia, Finland, and Scandinavia, where the berries are preserved in water or sugar and used as vitamin C during the winter. Lingonberries are traditionally made into a compote and served with reindeer meat (in Sweden and Norway) or with pork (in Denmark). Lingonberries have also been traditionally used as a dye for wool and cotton.

GROWING INFORMATION: Lingonberries are evergreen and keep their leaves during the cold northern winters. Preferring moist, cool summers, cold-hardy lingonberries do not grow well in areas with hot summers. Berries are harvested in the autumn.

THINGS TO BE AWARE OF: Lingonberry leaves have been shown to affect fertility in men; avoid using them if you are trying to conceive.

STEPHANIE'S FAVORITE USES: I love juicing lingonberries and also enjoy them "the Scandinavian way"—cooked into a sauce to accompany pork or meatballs and new potatoes.

MULBERRIES

NUTRITION PROFILE

PER SERVING: fresh (140 g)

BACKGROUND: These dark nubby fruits—which look a bit like blackberries—are native to China, where they serve a dual purpose: Their leaves are the only food that silkworms eat, making them an essential player in the silk industry. But they also have an established role in traditional Chinese medicine, where they have been used for thousands of years to treat heart disease, anemia, arthritis, and diabetes. In Europe and North America, they are often made into wine, juice, and preserves, as well as eaten fresh or dried.

CALORIES: 60

FIBER: This important nutrient offers a range of health benefits that include helping your body control blood sugar levels and promoting a sense of fullness after eating. A serving of mulberries provides 2.4 g of fiber.

VITAMIN C: You'll get 51 mg of vitamin C in a cup (140 g) of mulberries. This vitamin is essential in creating collagen, which is required for healthy cartilage and skin.

VITAMIN K: This nutrient helps control the thickness of your blood, ensuring that it will clot if you are injured. A serving of mulberries has 10.9 mcg of vitamin K.

IRON: In one serving of mulberries, there are 2.6 mg of iron, which helps store and transport oxygen via blood.

POTASSIUM: This essential mineral helps control blood pressure and reduces the risk of heart disease. A serving of mulberries offers 272 mg of potassium.

RIBOFLAVIN: Also called vitamin B_2, riboflavin defends your body against free radicals that damage your cells and contribute to aging. A cup of mulberries boasts 141 mcg of riboflavin.

ROLE IN SUPPORTING HEALTH

LOWERS BLOOD CHOLESTEROL LEVELS: Researchers from Chung Shan Medical University Hospital, Taichung, Taiwan, studied the effect of mulberry extract on rabbits that had high blood cholesterol levels. In the study, half of the rabbits received mulberry extract; the other half did not. At the end of ten days, the rabbits that received the mulberry extract experienced a 42 percent to 63 percent reduction of atherosclerosis in the aorta. The study was published in the August 2005 issue of *Food Chemistry*.

LOWERS BLOOD GLUCOSE LEVELS: One of the traditional medicinal uses of mulberries, and their leaves, is to help treat diabetes. In a study published in the 2007 issue of the *Journal of Agricultural and Food Chemistry*, researchers from Nippon Medical School, Tokyo, Japan, gave healthy volunteers a drink made with 0.8 or 1.2 g food-grade mulberry leaf powder or a placebo, followed by 50 g of sucrose. Plasma glucose and insulin were determined before, and 30 to 180 minutes after, the volunteers drank the mulberry solution and sucrose. The results? After drinking either of the mulberry leaf solutions, test subjects showed lowered blood sugar levels.

SUPPORTS PARKINSON'S DISEASE PATIENTS: Mulberries are a traditional remedy in Asia for Parkinson's disease, which is characterized by both the loss of dopaminergic neurons in the brain and increased oxidative stress on brain cells. A study performed by scientists from Kyung Hee University, Seoul, South Korea, published in the 2010 issue of the *British Journal of Nutrition*, looked at the role of mulberries on individuals with Parkinson's disease. Brain cells affected with Parkinson's disease that were treated with mulberry extract showed reduced concentrations of the disease as well as lower inflammation and oxidative stress.

REDUCES CANCEROUS TUMORS: In a study done on cancerous tissue, researchers from Dongguk University, Gyeongju, South Korea, found that when treated with mulberry extract, cancer cells extracted from cancerous tumors shrunk and even died. When mice with cancerous tumors received oral mulberry extract, tumors also shrunk. The study was published in the 2010 issue of *Nutrition and Cancer*.

GENERAL INFORMATION ABOUT MULBERRIES

Mulberries are available fresh and frozen. Because berries stop ripening the moment they are picked, opt for already-ripe, brightly colored fruits that show no signs of weepiness, mold, or moisture. If you purchase frozen berries, select unsweetened whole berries.

STORAGE: Do not wash mulberries until the moment you want to use them. Mulberries are highly perishable and should be stored (unwashed) for no more than two days before you use them. To store the berries, remove any weepy, smashed, or moldy fruit and store the remaining, unblemished fruit in a dry, shallow container with a paper towel or clean dishtowel over the fruit. Tightly cover the container and place it on a lower shelf or, ideally, in the produce drawer, of your refrigerator. If you cannot use the berries within a couple days, place the container in the freezer for up to six months.

USAGE: When you are ready to use your berries, gently wash them with cool water. It's important to be gentle so you don't break the berries. Some people place berries in a colander and submerge it into a container or sink filled with cold water, then allow the berries to drip dry. You can also mist the berries with a gentle stream of water. Pat them dry, if necessary, and use them immediately after washing.

BOTANICAL BACKGROUND: Mulberries come in red, black, pink, and white varieties. The tree is a member of the Moraceae family, comprised of about fifteen species of usually deciduous trees growing in Asia, North America, and Europe.

HISTORY: Because mulberry trees are necessary for silk production, they became one of the most important trees in ancient civilizations, planted all along the Silk Road that went from their native China to northern Africa, the Middle East, and Europe. The silk industry even hit North America, where the British Crown required colonists to grow silkworms and produce silk for the Crown. The tree's berries were used for dye and a medicine that was prescribed for everything from diabetes to constipation. The berries were also eaten out of hand as a food or cooked with meats.

GROWING INFORMATION: Mulberries can grow wild or cultivated and are popular yard trees in North America and Europe. They enjoy sunny locales with temperate climates and, depending on the variety, can tolerate low to heavy rain. Harvest is usually spring through autumn.

THINGS TO BE AWARE OF: Male mulberry trees are banned in some North American communities because of their heavy pollen production. Interestingly, the female mulberry tree is considered allergen-free and "sucks in" pollen produced by male trees as well as dust from the air.

STEPHANIE'S FAVORITE USES: I love mulberries cooked into a sauce and draped over chicken, fish, and waffles—or even stirred into a glass of sparkling water.

MULBERRIES: DID YOU KNOW?

- Mulberry silk is the softest and most valuable of all silks.
- Mulberry trees sometimes change from one sex to another.

RASPBERRIES

NUTRITION PROFILE

PER SERVING: (125 g)

BACKGROUND: One of the world's favorite berries, raspberries are ranked in the United States as the third most popular berry, right behind strawberries and blueberries. Versatile, nutritious, and delicious, these sweet-tart red berries are "aggregate fruits." This means that each berry is actually composed of many small individual fruits that come from multiple ovaries in a single flower. In the case of a raspberry, those small individual fruits are the little juicy spheres that make up the structure of the raspberry. They are also called drupelets, and each one has its own seed.

CALORIES: 64

FIBER: One serving of raspberries provides 7.99 g of fiber to help keep your digestive tract healthy, lower blood cholesterol, and help prevent colorectal cancer.

OMEGA-3 FATTY ACIDS: These help lower the risk of heart disease, support joint health, improve the skin, and support brain health by reducing the risk of depression and dementia. A serving of raspberries provides about 0.15 g of omega-3 fatty acids.

VITAMIN C: This water-soluble nutrient acts as an antioxidant, helping protect cells from the damage caused by free radicals, natural by-products of biochemical reactions in the body, including ordinary metabolic processes and immune system responses. Free radical–generating substances can be found in the food we eat, the drugs and medicines we take, the air we breathe, and the water we drink. A serving of raspberries provides 32.23 mg of vitamin C.

VITAMIN E: Another antioxidant, vitamin E helps keep the brain healthy and protects cells from damage caused by free radicals. A serving of raspberries provides 1.07 mg of the nutrient.

VITAMIN K: This important nutrient plays a vital role in blood clotting and helps prevent excessive bleeding. Researchers are currently looking into how the vitamin can help prevent and lessen bone loss. A serving of raspberries provides 9.59 mcg of vitamin K.

COPPER: Dietary copper is helpful in the production of red blood cells and assists with our sense of taste. A serving of raspberries provides about 0.11 mg of copper.

FOLATE: Also known as vitamin B_9, or folic acid, folate helps the body make new cells. A serving of raspberries provides 25.83 mcg of folate.

MANGANESE: You'll get 0.82 mg of manganese, a mineral that helps you metabolize both fat and protein, from raspberries. Manganese also supports both the immune and nervous systems and promotes stable blood sugar levels.

MAGNESIUM: One serving of raspberries delivers about 27.06 mg of magnesium, a mineral responsible for many biochemical functions in the body, including regulating the heart's rhythm and supporting the function of nerve cells. Magnesium is a major electrolyte that helps maintain proper fluid levels in the body and regulates muscle function.

PANTOTHENIC ACID: Known as vitamin B_5, pantothenic acid is essential to a wide range of chemical reactions in the body that sustain life. One serving of raspberries offers 0.4 mg of the nutrient.

POTASSIUM: You'll get 185.73 mg of potassium from a serving of raspberries. This essential mineral, a major electrolyte, helps maintain proper fluid levels in the body and regulate muscle function. It also plays an important role in nerve function and blood pressure.

ROLE IN SUPPORTING HEALTH

HELPS FIGHT BREAST CANCER: About one in eight women in the United States will develop breast cancer over her lifetime, and currently there are more than 2 million breast-cancer survivors, many of whom are concerned with recurrence. Cancer-fighting ellagic acid appears in high amounts in strawberries, raspberries, and blackberries. In animal and test-tube studies—such as one performed by researchers at Shahid Beheshti University of Medical Sciences, Tehran, Iran, and published in the September 2015 issue of *Redox Biology*—these compounds have been shown to stop the growth of breast, colon, and esophageal cancer cells.

KILLS DANGEROUS BACTERIA: A study done in 2005 by a research team from the University of Helsinki, Finland, found that the anthocyanins in raspberries greatly slowed the growth of two fast-growing and health-compromising bacteria, *Proteus mirabilis*, an easily spread bacteria that infects the intestinal and urinary tracts, and *Klebsiella oxytoca*, a drug-resistant bacteria that is often found in hospitals and nursing homes. This study was published in the April 2005 issue of *Journal of Applied Microbiology*.

KEEPS OUR BRAINS YOUNG: In an article in the March 2012 issue of *American Chemical Society*, two scientists—Marshal G. Miller and Barbara Shukitt-Hale—analyzed research data from cellular, animal, and human studies on brain health. They found that high amounts of antioxidants in raspberries and other berries can help prevent or lessen the severity of dementia, Alzheimer's disease, and other brain conditions when eaten weekly. The two researchers also reported that berry fruits change the way neurons in the brain communicate. These changes in signaling can prevent inflammation in the brain that contributes to neuron damage and improve both motor control and cognition.

REDUCES INFLAMMATION IN THE BODY: Inflammation causes chronic pain and disease, which is why the medical world spends so much energy searching for and talking about anti-inflammatories. A research team from Andong National University in the Republic of Korea found a connection between a natural chemical in the raspberry (and other plants) called raspberry ketone (responsible for the fruit's heavenly aroma) and the reduction of inflammation in the body, thanks to an inflammation-inhibiting enzyme. The results were published in the September 2010 issue of *Food and Chemical Toxicology*.

SUPPORTS HEART HEALTH: In 2007, researchers from Pacific Agri-Food Research Centre, British Columbia, Canada, investigated a range of fruits and berries for the level and activity of anthocyanins, a phytochemical in raspberries and other deeply colored fruit. Anythocyanins behave like natural ibuprofen, helping the body block signals that cause pain and inflammation in the heart and in other organs. This review was published in the 2007 issue of the Italian journal *Annali dell'Istituto Superiore di Sanità*.

HELPS MAKE IT EASIER TO SEE IN DIM LIGHT: Researchers at the Atlantic Food and Horticulture Research Centre in Canada examined the effects of anthocyanins in raspberries on vision. They found that anthocyanins and other phytonutrients in raspberries interact directly with rhodopsin, the photosensitive pigment in the eye that helps you see in dim light. The verdict, published in the April 2010 issue of *Journal of Agricultural and Food Chemistry*, is that anthocyanins protect the eye tissue from cell death.

GENERAL INFORMATION ABOUT RASPBERRIES

Raspberries are available fresh and frozen. Because raspberries stop ripening the moment they are picked, opt for already-ripe, brightly colored fruits that show no signs of weepiness, mold, or moisture. If you purchase frozen berries, choose unsweetened whole berries or unsweetened raspberry puree.

STORAGE: Do not wash raspberries until the moment you want to use them. Raspberries are highly perishable and should be stored (again, unwashed) no more than two days before enjoying. Remove any weepy, smashed, or moldy berries, and store the remaining unblemished fruit in a dry, shallow container with a paper towel or clean dishtowel over the fruit. Tightly cover the container and place it on a lower shelf or, ideally, in the produce drawer, of your refrigerator. If you cannot use the berries within a couple days, place the container in the freezer for up to six months.

USAGE: When you are ready to use the berries, gently wash them with cool water. It's important to be gentle so you don't break the berries. Some people place berries in a colander and submerge it in a container or sink filled with cold water and then allow the berries to drip dry. You can also clean the berries under a gentle stream of water. Pat them dry if necessary and use them immediately after washing.

BOTANICAL BACKGROUND: Raspberries are members of the rose family. There are about 200 different varieties of raspberries, both wild and cultivated, grown throughout Europe, North America, Central America, South America, New Zealand, Australia, and northern Asia. Most raspberries are a soft red color, but there are yellow, white, lavender, and deep plum-colored raspberries, all with a similar taste and nutrient profile. Any of these can be used in the recipes in this book that call for raspberries.

HISTORY: Wild raspberries were first cultivated throughout Europe, North America, and northern Asia, where they were used as an important seasonal food source. When people learned how to preserve berries through drying, they began to pulverize and blend the dried fruit into mixtures of meat and nuts for winter consumption. Throughout history, we have used both raspberries and raspberry leaves as medicine. The berries have been eaten to treat constipation and help heal psoriasis and eczema. The leaves—which are rich in magnesium, potassium, iron, and B vitamins—are brewed into an herbal tea that is consumed for nausea, leg cramps, menstrual cramps, heavy periods, and strengthening the uterus in preparation for pregnancy.

GROWING INFORMATION: Raspberries grow on thorny, woody stems known as canes, which grown tangled into brambles. Raspberries prefer fertile soil and a bit of coolness during the fall, winter, and spring. They typically bear fruit during the summer, although there are varieties that are harvested in late spring or early autumn.

THINGS TO BE AWARE OF: People following a low oxalate diet may want to speak to their health-care provider before enjoying large amounts of raspberries. Raspberries contain 15 to 25 mg of oxalates per 3.5 ounces (100 g).

STEPHANIE'S FAVORITE USES: Instead of putting sugary store-bought raspberry jam or jelly on your next PB&J sandwich, simply mash some whole berries and spread them over the peanut butter. Delicious. I also love raspberries pureed and stirred into chia pudding, liquefied with hot coconut milk for a warm fruity beverage, and folded whole into cornbread or yellow cake batter.

STRAWBERRIES

NUTRITION PROFILE

PER SERVING: (145 g)

BACKGROUND: Strawberries are the most popular fruit in the United States. Unlike brambleberries—such as raspberries and blackberries—which are often gathered from wild bushes and enjoy a reputation as "berries for the masses," strawberries have long been considered a luxury fruit for the wealthy. These jewel-toned fruits have retained their high-end reputation. Perfectly shaped, long-stemmed strawberries are sold by the dozen—ideal for dipping in chocolate.

CALORIES: 46

FIBER: A 1-cup (165 g) serving of strawberries provides 2.88 g of fiber, a nutrient that helps with digestion by adding bulk to the stool, which in turn helps move food through the digestive tract while

SALMONBERRIES

This wild-growing fruit is native to the Pacific Northwest region of North America. Salmonberries look a bit like raspberries, except they are smaller, more golden in color, and contain a white core that sometimes falls out upon picking. So how do they taste? Sour. Salmonberries contain small amounts of vitamins A and B_6 and a moderate amount of vitamin C, plus anti-inflammatory phytonutrients. Enjoy them raw or toss a few into a fruit smoothie.

"cleaning" the interior wall of the large intestine. Fiber has been shown to help with weight loss by creating a feeling of fullness, which discourages overeating.

OMEGA-3 FATTY ACIDS: Vital for normal cell development and growth, this nutrient complex also helps keep the cardiovascular and nervous systems healthy. A serving of strawberries provides about 0.09 g.

VITAMIN B_6: This vitamin is involved in brain development and immune function in utero and during infancy. A serving of strawberries will give you 0.07 mg.

VITAMIN C: This powerful antioxidant can help prevent and lessen the duration of viral illnesses, stimulate collagen production for fast wound healing, and help prevent a variety of diseases, from cancer to cataracts. A serving of strawberries will provide 84.67 mg of this nutrient.

BIOTIN: Breaking down fats and carbohydrates and helping keep hair, skin, and nails healthy are some of the work this B-family vitamin does in the body. A serving of strawberries provides 1.58 mcg of biotin.

COPPER: Dietary copper helps in the production of red blood cells and assists with our sense of taste. A serving of strawberries provides about 0.07 mg of copper.

FOLATE: This B vitamin is naturally present in many foods. The body needs folate to make DNA and other genetic material as well as to help cells divide. A serving of strawberries provides 34.56 mcg.

IODINE: The thyroid needs iodine to make hormones. A serving of strawberries will provide 12.96 mcg of iodine.

MANGANESE: One serving of strawberries offers 0.56 mg of manganese, a mineral that the body needs to process cholesterol, carbohydrates, and protein.

MAGNESIUM: This mineral is required for the proper growth and maintenance of bones. It is also needed for the correct functioning of nerves, muscles, and many other parts of the body. A serving of strawberries delivers about 18.72 mg of magnesium.

PHOSPHORUS: After calcium, phosphorus is the second most abundant mineral in the body. It helps create strong bones and teeth. A serving of strawberries will provide about 34.56 mg of phosphorus.

POTASSIUM: This mineral is essential for fluid balance within your cells. It is also necessary for proper heart function and muscle growth. You'll get 220.32 mg of potassium from a serving of strawberries.

ROLE IN SUPPORTING HEALTH

HELPS SAFEGUARD MENTAL ACUITY: Women who eat about two servings of strawberries or one serving of blueberries a week experienced less mental decline over time than peers who went without these nutrition powerhouses, according to research published in the April 2012 issue of *Annals of Neurology*. In the study, researchers reviewed data collected between 1995 and 2001 from 16,010 women over age seventy, as part of the *Nurses' Health Study*. Individuals with the highest berry intake postponed cognitive decline by about two and a half years. Berries' antioxidant levels are the secret.

REGULATES BLOOD SUGAR LEVELS: In a study published in the September 2011 issue of the *British Journal of Nutrition*, twenty-four overweight individuals were fed a high-carbohydrate meal, then given a drink made of strawberries or a placebo drink. Subjects who consumed the strawberry drink had lower blood sugar levels as well as lower post-meal blood-inflammation markers than those who received the placebo drink.

PROTECTS AGAINST INFLAMMATORY DISEASES: Researchers at the Harvard School of Public Health studying the value of strawberries found that women who consumed sixteen or more fresh or frozen strawberries per week were 14 percent less likely than non-strawberry eaters to have elevated levels of the protein in their blood, an indication of an inflammatory disease, such as a marrow disorder, multiple myeloma, arthritis, human immunodeficiency virus (HIV), amyloidosis or other chronic inflammatory conditions. This study was published in the August 2007 issue of the *Journal of the American College of Nutrition*.

PROTECTS AGAINST CANCER: In a study published in the August 2007 issue of *Neurobiology of Aging*, rats whose brains were artificially aged through radiation were supplemented with 2 percent strawberry extract. These rats were able to retard and even reverse age-related changes in the brain compared to a control group that did not receive the strawberry extract.

HELPS LOWER BLOOD CHOLESTEROL LEVELS: In a study at St. Michael's Hospital, Toronto, Canada, twenty-eight individuals with elevated cholesterol levels were given either 65 g (2 slices) of oat bran bread daily or 454 g (3 cups) of strawberries a day. After one month, both groups had lower cholesterol levels; however, the strawberry group had cholesterol levels that were two points lower and also enjoyed an increase in antioxidant intake, which reduced oxidative damage. The study was published in the December 2008 issue of *Metabolism*.

GENERAL INFORMATION ABOUT STRAWBERRIES

Strawberries are available fresh and frozen. Because berries stop ripening the moment they are picked, opt for already-ripe, brightly colored fruits that show no signs of weepiness, mold, or moisture. If you purchase frozen berries, select unsweetened whole berries.

Note: Most commercially available strawberries are crunchy and unripe, so I prefer to buy them from farmers' markets or grow my own. They are best enjoyed in season. If you have overly firm, insipid-tasting berries, slice and dress them with a bit of lemon juice, a few grains of salt, or a tiny bit of sweetener and a splash of vanilla extract. This will greatly improve their taste.

STORAGE: Do not wash strawberries until the moment you want to use them. Strawberries are highly perishable and should be stored unwashed. Remove any weepy, smashed, or moldy berries as well as any leaves or stems (but don't core the berries). Store unblemished fruit in a dry, shallow container with a paper towel or clean dishtowel over the fruit. Tightly cover the container and place it on a lower shelf or, ideally, in the produce drawer, of your refrigerator for no more than two days before use. If you cannot use the berries within a couple days, place the container in the freezer for up to six months.

USAGE: Gently rinse the berries with cool water and quickly cut out the core at the stem end. Pat them dry if necessary and use immediately.

BOTANICAL BACKGROUND: Strawberries belong to the Rosaceae family, along with apples, peaches, and yes, roses. Scientists don't know for certain when or where strawberries first appeared, but there are around 600 varieties of wild and cultivated berries that grow in a wide range of habitats.

HISTORY: Strawberries have grown in the wild for thousands and thousands of years. After numerous attempts to tame one or more of the hundreds of varieties of wild strawberries, French growers succeeded in 1714, when they crossed a European strawberry with a wild strawberry brought back from South America by early explorers. The rest is delicious history.

GROWING INFORMATION: When planted in rich, moist, but well-drained soil and given plenty of sunlight, strawberry plants will bear fruit heavily for three or so years before gradually slowing down. While most plants grow from seeds, strawberry plants propogate from runners—long stems that grow away from the plant and take root nearby. This means that a strawberry bed can grow and spread almost exponentially unless you periodically prune the runners before they can take root and grow new plants.

THINGS TO BE AWARE OF: When grown conventionally, strawberries tend to have pesticide residue. According to the Environmental Working Group's 2015 report, *Shopper's Guide to Pesticides in Produce*™, conventionally grown strawberries are fourth on the list of the most highly contaminated fruits and vegetables in the United States. Purchasing organic strawberries, or growing your own, ensures you get the important nutrients that strawberries have to offer without any potentially harmful chemicals.

STEPHANIE'S FAVORITE USES: I love strawberries sliced and dressed with a dollop of Whipped Coconut Cream (see page 150) or with a few shavings of dark chocolate and a dusting of chopped walnuts. I also enjoy adding a few strawberries to my juicer when I make my morning green drink.

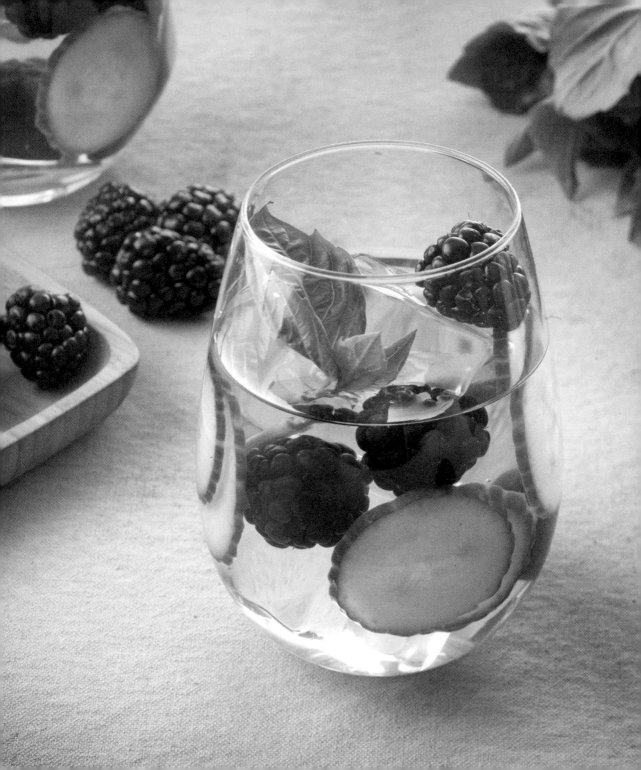

CHAPTER 3

DRINK YOUR BERRIES

With their bright, sunny taste, berries make a natural addition to drinks of all kinds, from frosty shakes to smoothies to slushies and coolers—even hot drinks such as caffeinated and herbal teas. And yes, while I love the yummy taste of berries as much as the next person, the nutritionist in me adores the nutritional punch berries bring to drinks of all kinds—notably fiber and a host of antioxidants, from vitamin C to polyphenols—which helps boost your immune system, prevent cancer, help heart function, and so much more.

COOLERS

SPARKLING BERRY COOLER

MAKES 4 1-CUP (250 ML) SERVINGS

People love their fruit juice, often believing that it is healthier than it really is because it comes from fruit. Although it's true that fruit juice has plenty of vitamins, it is also true that it contains plentiful amounts of fructose, which can contribute to diabetes, elevated blood sugar levels, fat around the midsection, and obesity. Before you go running for the diet soda, let me give you a way to enjoy fruit juice in moderation, with this easy-to-make cooler. I've used unsweetened cranberry juice or raspberry juice in this recipe, but you can swap in any berry juice you'd like, from blueberry to elderberry. Just make sure you use unsweetened, 100 percent juice.

2 cups (475 ml) unsweetened cranberry or raspberry juice (or a combination)

2 cups (475 ml) sparkling water

2 tablespoons lime juice

Optional: Ice

Optional: ½ cup (125 g) fresh or frozen raspberries or other berries for garnish

Optional: Lime slices for garnish

1. In a large pitcher, combine the juice, sparkling water, and lime juice.

2. Divide among four glasses (with or without ice). Garnish with frozen berries and lime slices if desired.

OPPOSITE: **Blackberry Cucumber Water, page 55**

SPARKLY WATERS:
YOUR CHOICES

Have you ever wondered what the difference is between mineral, sparkling, carbonated, and tonic water? If you're equally mystified by club soda and seltzer, this primer is for you!

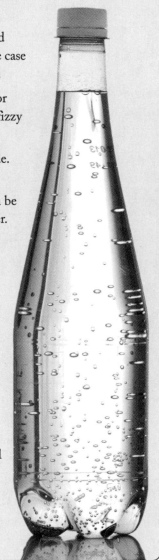

- **CARBONATED WATER** is a generic term for any water-based, unflavored liquid that contains bubbles. These bubbles can occur naturally (in the case of mineral water) or they can be made artificially with carbon dioxide.

- **SPARKLING WATER** is the same as carbonated water; the definition for carbonated water also describes sparkling water. (Bubbly water and fizzy water are interchangeable with sparkling or carbonated water.)

- **SELTZER** is carbonated water that is made bubbly with carbon dioxide. It contains no other ingredients.

- **MINERAL WATER** comes from a mineral spring. While this water can be flat, most people use the term to refer to naturally "carbonated" water. The US Food and Drug Administration defines mineral water as water "containing not less than 250 parts per million (ppm) total dissolved solids that originates from a geologically and physically protected underground water source."

- **SPRING WATER** is flat or naturally sparkling water originating from an underground source that contains less than 250 ppm dissolved minerals.

- **CLUB SODA** is artificially carbonated water to which salt (table salt, baking soda, and/or potassium) has been added to mimic the flavors of naturally occurring mineral water.

- **TONIC WATER** isn't really water. It's a lightly sweetened drink containing carbonated water and quinine. Quinine is an antimalarial compound that was originally added to tonic water for its medicinal effects, but it is now added in trace quantities for its unique bitter flavor. (None of the recipes in the section should be used with tonic water. Who needs the artificial sugar?)

STRAWBERRY BASIL SODA

MAKES 2 2-CUP (475 ML) SERVINGS

This sophisticated drink is refreshing and very grown-up. It is also a great way to use overripe or super-ripe berries, although you can substitute raspberries or blackberries if you don't have any strawberries on hand.

- 4 tablespoons lemon juice
- 1 tablespoon raw sugar
- 10 basil leaves
- 10 small strawberries (or 6 large strawberries, quartered) plus 1 thin slice of strawberry to garnish each glass
- 1 pinch kosher salt
- 1½ cups (350 ml) sparkling water
- Ice cubes

1. In a pitcher, combine the lemon juice, raw sugar, basil, whole strawberries, and salt. Muddle the ingredients with a muddler or the handle of a wooden spoon until sugar dissolves.

2. Add the sparkling water and stir until ingredients are blended.

3. Add the ice cubes to two tall glasses.

4. Strain soda through cheesecloth or a sieve into prepared glasses. Garnish with strawberry slices if desired.

BLACKBERRY CUCUMBER WATER

MAKES ABOUT 4 1-CUP (250 ML) SERVINGS

This refreshing beverage is adult (read: civilized), though you could share it with the kids. It's best sipped while seated outdoors on a porch, deck, or wherever you want to enjoy the summery flavors of this refreshing drink.

- 1 6-ounce package (170 g) of blackberries (about 1 generous cup)
- 1 cup (120 g) thinly sliced cucumber (if desired, peel before slicing)
- 4 to 5 Thai basil leaves (or use regular basil)
- 4 cups (1 L) sparkling water

1. Add the berries, cucumber, and Thai basil to a pitcher. Top with sparkling water and stir well. Cover and chill for at least two hours to allow flavors to blend.

2. For easier pouring and drinking, remove the basil before serving.

WHAT DOES MUDDLE MEAN?

Muddle is a word used often in cocktail culture. It comes from the Old English word for wallowing in mud. What it means in the drink world, however, is to smash ingredients with a blunt instrument to release flavors.

GINGER BERRY SWITCHEL

MAKES ABOUT 4 1-CUP (250 ML) SERVINGS

A switchel is an old-fashioned vinegar-based drink used to quench thirst. It reminds me a bit of the commercial kombucha drinks that are so popular today.

1   5-inch/12.5-cm piece fresh ginger (about 6 ounces/170g)

½   cup (125 ml) apple cider vinegar

3   tablespoons pure maple syrup

1   tablespoon lemon juice

½   cup (60 g) berries of your choice (I particularly like currants, raspberries, or blackberries; blueberries don't work as well as other berries.)

4   cups (1 L) sparkling or flat water

1. Pass the ginger through a juicer (you should have about ⅓ cup/80 ml). Or, you can grate the ginger on a box grater, gather it up in a square of cheesecloth, and squeeze shavings over a bowl to catch ginger juice. (You'll probably have less than a ⅓ cup/80 ml, but that's just fine.)

2. Combine the ginger juice, vinegar, maple syrup, and lemon juice in a large pitcher and stir until maple syrup is dissolved.

ICY BERRY CUBES

Berry ice cubes add a delightful touch of whimsy to summer drinks and are a fun way to flavor juices and waters. Plus, they are super easy to make.

Grab an ice cube tray or ice molds and place 1 or 2 berries in each indentation. Fill each indentation with water, lemon water, lemonade, or fruit juice. Make sure each berry is fully submerged. Leave the mold in the freezer until the ingredients are frozen. Use the frozen cubes or molds in any drink you desire, from tap water or seltzer, to fruit juice, to champagne or cocktails. (My kids like to crunch on these cubes sans beverage.)

Note: When I make Icy Berry Cubes, I like to use currants, raspberries, and blackberries best. Strawberries can get a little spongy when frozen, mulberries are a bit seedy, and blueberries, though they look beautiful, don't flavor drinks well thanks to their thick skins.

3. Add the berries and muddle or leave whole.

4. Refrigerate until chilled.

5. To serve, dilute with water to taste and ladle switchel into ice-filled glasses.

SMOOTHIES

SUPERFOOD PURPLE SMOOTHIE

MAKES 1 3-CUP (700 ML) SERVING

I know you don't really need a recipe to make a smoothie, right? You just toss a bunch of fruit and veggies in a blender with your choice of liquids and blend, blend, blend. But sometimes an interesting recipe comes along that makes you expand your ideas about what's possible for the humble smoothie. This intriguing recipe is exactly what I'm talking about. Not only is it unusual, but also it's loaded with superfoods in the form of blueberries (or blackberries), beets, and coconut.

- *1 cup (155 g) frozen blueberries (or blackberries)*
- *1 small raw beet, peeled and grated or chopped very fine*
- *1½ cups (350 ml) coconut milk*
- *Optional: ½ tablespoon coconut oil*
- *Optional: Squirt of lemon or lime juice*

1. Place all ingredients in a high-powered blender, such as a Vitamix® or Blendtec®, blend until smooth, and enjoy! If using a standard blender, you'll have to blend a while to get a smooth texture.

RASPBERRY CELERY SMOOTHIE

MAKES 1 2-CUP (500 ML) SERVING

Yes, I know this one sounds weird. But it is refreshing, fruity (without being overly-sweet), incredibly detoxifying (thanks to the celery), and super for your immune system (those raspberries—and the mangoes—are filled with phytonutrients, fiber, and vitamin C). For something different, replace the celery with a handful of baby spinach. I've also tried this with blackberries and cranberries, which, while lovely, require a bit of extra blending.

- *1 cup (125 g) fresh or frozen raspberries*
- *1 banana (try a frozen banana), peeled*
- *½ cup (85 g) fresh or frozen mango, chopped*
- *1 cup (250 ml) coconut milk (or use hemp, almond, or another nut or seed milk)*
- *3 stalks of celery (I like the tender inner stalks.)*
- *Optional: A few ice cubes (You won't need ice if using any frozen ingredients.)*

1. Place all ingredients in a high-powered blender, such as a Vitamix or Blendtec, and blend until smooth. If using a standard blender, you'll have to blend a while to get a smooth texture.

HOMEMADE BERRY SYRUP

MAKES ONE CUP (250 ML) OF SYRUP

Berry syrup is easy to make and you get the benefit of fresh taste without high-fructose corn syrup, cane sugar, and artificial colorings and flavorings.

- 2 cups (245 g) berries (Mulberries, strawberries, blueberries, raspberries, and blackberries are good choices. Cranberries won't work here—you'll have sauce.)
- 1 cup (250 ml) water
- 1 cup (145 g) coconut sugar, Grade B maple syrup (the finished product won't taste "maple-y"), or unfiltered honey
- ½ to 1 tablespoon lemon juice

1. If using larger berries, such as strawberries, slice them in half first.

2. Place all the ingredients in a medium saucepot and bring to a rolling boil.

3. Cover and reduce heat to low, and simmer for ten to twelve minutes, until berries have broken down and the liquid has begun to thicken.

4. Remove the lid and allow the mixture to cool a bit. Pour the mixture into a blender or food processor, or leave in the pot and use an immersion blender. Blend until the berries are liquefied. For a clear syrup, pour the liquid through a strainer or cheesecloth. Pour the mixture—strained or unstrained—back into the pot.

5. Leaving the pot uncovered, simmer the mixture for five to six minutes more, until reduced to about 1 cup (250 ml).

6. Remove from the heat and stir in the lemon juice.

7. Allow the liquid to cool before decanting to a tightly sealed jar. The syrup will keep for several weeks refrigerated.

8. To use, pour one tablespoon (more or less) into a glass of seltzer or sparkling wine, or use it with your favorite milk to make "berry milk." The syrup can also be poured over waffles and pancakes and used as a flavoring for just about anything.

BLUEBERRY-CABBAGE POWER JUICE

MAKES ABOUT 2 1-CUP (250 ML) SERVINGS

I have to admit that I don't juice a lot of berries. Although they taste amazing when juiced—either alone or blended with other fruit or veggie juices—they don't yield much liquid and, because of their seeds and fiber, they really gum up a juicer. Blueberries and cranberries, with all the pectin they contain, are especially problematic. Having said that, I do love their taste, so I will often toss a few berries into a juice. In this recipe, the anticancer fighting power of cabbage pairs with detoxifying cucumber and blueberries or blackberries to create a lovely purple juice. I love this as an afternoon pick-me-up.

- 2 *cups (140 g) sliced or chopped red cabbage*
- 2 *large cucumbers, peeled if desired, and sliced in half or quarters horizontally*
- 1 *lemon, peel removed and sliced into quarters*
- ½ *cup (75 g) blueberries or blackberries*
- 1 *large Granny Smith (or other tart variety) apple, cut into eighths*

1. Working in this order, push the cabbage, cucumber, lemon, berries, and apple through your juicer according to the manufacturer's directions.

2. Drink the juice within twenty minutes of making it in order to benefit the most from the nutrients. If you have to make this juice ahead, add the juice of an entire extra lemon to help preserve the vitamin content and color of the drink.

NO JUICER? USE YOUR BLENDER!

Remove cores, stems, and seeds from ingredients (I usually leave them on when using a juicer, but you must remove them when using a blender). Chop all ingredients. Place the softest and juiciest of your ingredients in the blender with ¼ cup (50 ml) of water (or another healthy liquid of your choice), and process until liquefied. Add the sturdier ingredients and another ¼ cup (50 ml) of water and process until liquefied. Then, add the remaining ingredients; blend until liquefied. If you have a high-powered blender, such as a Blendtec or Vitamix, you can easily process the mixture until ingredients are a smooth liquid, adding more water if necessary to get the desired texture. If you have a standard blender, you may want to strain the liquid through a cheesecloth or a sieve.

MORNING GLORY JUICE

MAKES 2 ½-CUP (125 ML) SERVINGS

I call this morning glory juice because it has many of the same ingredients as the famous morning glory muffins I used to enjoy. This is a yummy, pretty juice that is great for strengthening the immune system. If your family dislikes juice, share this one. I promise it will win them over to juicing.

6 *strawberries, hulled*

1 *large cucumber, peeled and cut into chunks*

½ *lemon, peeled and cut into quarters*

1 *large Granny Smith (or other tart variety) apple, cut into eighths*

2 *medium carrots*

1. Working in this order, push the strawberries, cucumber, lemon, apple, and carrots through your juicer according to the manufacturer's directions.

2. Drink within twenty minutes to benefit from the highest nutrient content. If you have to make this juice ahead of time, add the juice of an entire extra lemon to help preserve the vitamin content and color.

WINTER BERRY JUICE

MAKES 2 ½-CUP (125 ML) SERVINGS

A lot of juice aficionados stop juicing in the winter, when fresh fruit and vegetables are more limited. Not me! I turn my attention to warming combinations that feature fall and autumn produce. This one, with cranberries, carrots, apples, and ginger, is delicious and great for keeping you healthy and strong during the cold and flu season. Thanks to the cranberries, it can also help prevent urinary tract infections.

1 *cup (100 g) cranberries*

½ *lemon, peeled and quartered*

2 *apples (any kind) or pears (any kind)*

3 *carrots*

1 *1-inch (2½ cm) slice fresh ginger*

1. Working in this order, push the cranberries, lemon, apples (or pears), carrots, and ginger through your juicer according to the manufacturer's directions.

2. Drink within twenty minutes to benefit from the highest nutrient content. If you have to make this juice ahead of time, add the juice of an entire extra lemon to help preserve the vitamin content and color.

Unsweetened cranberry juice packs a powerful antioxidant punch and is great for helping to ward off viruses and preventing urinary tract infections, as well as lessening the symptoms and shortening the duration of established UTIs. However, cranberry juice isn't for everyone. If you have a history of kidney stones, you should avoid drinking cranberry juice. The most common type of kidney stone consists of calcium and oxalate, which are exacerbated by high-oxalate foods, such as cranberry juice. Even if you don't suffer from kidney stones, limit your consumption to no more than 4 cups daily for five or more days, because cranberry juice may increase your risk of kidney stones.

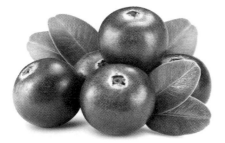

HOT TEAS

WHITE BERRY TEA

MAKES 2 1-CUP SERVINGS

White tea is harvested before the tea plant's leaves open fully, when the young buds are still covered by fine white hairs, hence the name "white" tea. Its light, delicate flavor pairs beautifully with berries of all types. Feel free to use fresh, dried, or frozen berries of your choice in this recipe.

2½ cups (600 ml) water

2 white tea teabags (or use 2 tablespoons of loose white tea)

12 berries of your choice (fresh, frozen, or dried)

Optional: 2 tablespoons unfiltered honey

Optional: 2 tablespoons lemon juice

1. In a small saucepot over medium heat, boil water. Add the tea bags and berries and turn off the heat. Allow to steep for two or three minutes.

2. Remove the tea bags; smash the berries a bit with the back of a fork or a potato masher.

3. Strain the liquid through a sieve or colander.

4. Stir in the honey and lemon juice if desired.

BERRY THERAPY

Berries offer remarkable immune-strengthening qualities, making them a favorite ingredient in many wellness preparations. The following recipes provide gentle, delicious ways to support your health every day.

CRANBERRY DRINK
MAKES 1 CUP (250 ML)

Growing up, I experienced frequents bouts of bronchitis and pneumonia. When I was in high school, my boyfriend's mother used to make this drink for me.

1 cup (250 ml) unsweetened cranberry juice

Optional: 1 cinnamon stick, 1 star anise, or 2 to 3 whole cloves

Optional: A few slices of lemon or orange

Optional: A drizzle of unfiltered raw honey

Add the juice to a small saucepot over low heat. Add some or all of the optional ingredients and heat until desired temperature. Strain before serving if desired.

ELDERBERRY SYRUP
MAKES ABOUT 2 CUPS (475 ML)

Elderberries have long been used for taming cold and flu symptoms by decreasing mucous production, providing vitamins A and C as well as bioflavonoids, and strengthening the immune system. This syrup is so delicious you may find yourself using it on pancakes, for a dessert sauce, or as a flavoring for seltzer.

½ cup (45 g) dried elderberries

3½ cups (825 ml) water

1   stick cinnamon or a couple whole cloves

1   slice fresh ginger

½ cup (70 g) coconut sugar

1. Place the elderberries, water, cloves, ginger, and coconut sugar in a small pot over medium heat. Bring to a boil. Reduce the heat to low and simmer the liquid for about thirty minutes.

2. Strain and discard the elderberries and spices. (You can blend the elderberries into a smoothie if desired.)

3. Once cool, pour the mixture into a clean glass jar. Refrigerate for up to two months.

4. Take 1 tablespoon daily during cold and flu season; take 2 or 3 tablespoons per day if you have a cold or flu. There are no side effects.

HAWTHORN BERRY TEA
MAKES ABOUT 3 CUPS (700 ML)

Traditionally, hawthorn berries have been used to prevent and treat heart conditions, including poor circulation, hypertension, inflammation, and high cholesterol. Several human and animal studies support the health benefits of hawthorn berries.

1 cup (115 g) hawthorn berries (or ½ cup/45 g dried berries)
3 cups (700 ml) water
½ to 1 cup (125 to 250 ml) unfiltered raw honey (to taste)

1. In a saucepot over medium heat, add water and hawthorne berries. Bring to a rolling boil. Reduce the heat to low and simmer for five minutes.

2. Turn the heat off and, using the back of a fork or a potato masher, mash the hawthorn berries until you just can't mash them anymore!

3. Strain the liquid, discarding the berries. Add the honey to the liquid, stirring until dissolved.

4. Pour the liquid into a dark, sealable glass jar or bottle and refrigerate for no more than three months. Use 1 tablespoon (or more) a day stirred into seltzer or hot or cold water. You can also enjoy it on waffles and pancakes or as a dessert sauce.

MULLED BERRY TEA

MAKES 6 1-CUP SERVINGS

This tastes a bit like the hot lemonade many of our grandmothers used to make for us when we were kids and had a cold, except this recipe for that warming beverage includes cranberry juice and tea—with a few raspberries thrown in for good measure. It is yummy and filled with antioxidants to help strengthen your immune system. If you have any tea leftover, chill it for an equally delicious libation.

- 1 cup (250 g) frozen raspberries, slightly thawed
- 2 cups (475 ml) brewed black tea
- 2 cups (475 ml) unsweetened cranberry juice
- 1 cup (250 ml) prepared lemonade
- ¼ cup (50 ml) water
- 3 whole allspice berries
- 1 lemon, thinly sliced

1. Add the raspberries to a large saucepot over low heat. Partially mash berries with a potato masher.

2. Stir in the tea, cranberry juice, lemonade, water, and allspice berries. Bring to a boil and reduce the heat.

3. Add the lemon slices and simmer uncovered for ten minutes. Strain and discard fruit pulp and spices.

4. Ladle into heatproof glass mugs or cups. Sweeten with your favorite natural sweetener if desired.

GOJI BERRIES: DID YOU KNOW?

- The young shoots and the leaves of the goji berry plant can be used as cooking greens.

- Many people harvest goji berries by laying a tarp on the ground and simply shaking the tree. Ripe fruit drops from the branches.

- Goji berry is not actually a berry—it's a fruit that belongs to the nightshade family. Famous cousins include the tomato, eggplant, potato, and tobacco.

- The majority of commercially produced goji berries come from the Ningxia region of north central China and the Xinjiang Uyghur autonomous region of western China, where the berries are grown on 100- to 1,000-acre plantations.

- The number of seeds in each goji berry varies widely, based on cultivar and fruit size, containing anywhere from ten to sixty tiny yellow seeds that are compressed within a curved embryo.

GOJI BERRY TEA

MAKES 1 1-CUP SERVING

This easy infusion, which is more of a blueprint than a recipe, lets you enjoy the immune-boosting benefits of the goji berry in a no-fuss, fun, delicious way. You can also make this tea with dried white mulberries, using the same directions and amounts of dried berries and boiling water.

1 to 2 tablespoons dried goji berries

1 cup (250 ml) or more boiling water

1. Add dried goji berries to the bottom of a teacup or mug. Pour boiling water over the berries, filling the cup.

2. Allow to steep for five minutes.

3. Remove the goji berries, sweeten as desired, and enjoy.

BERRY HERBAL TEA WITH ORANGE SLICES

MAKES 4 1-CUP SERVINGS

This berry herbal tea is a great caffeine-free option. My kids love it! Red Zinger®, an herbal tea based on hibiscus flowers, was introduced by Celestial Seasonings™ in 1972 and remains one of their best-sellers.

3 cups (700 ml) water

4 Red Zinger or hibiscus flower tea bags

1 orange, sliced in thin horizontal slices

1 cup (250 ml) unsweetened cranberry juice

1. Bring the water to a boil in a medium saucepot. Add the tea bags and orange slices.

2. Pour in the cranberry juice. Cover the saucepot, remove from the heat, and allow the tea to seep for three minutes.

3. Remove the tea bags and orange slices.

4. Ladle or pour the tea into six cups.

5. Leftovers may be chilled and enjoyed cold.

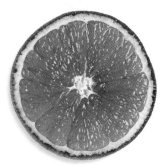

COLD TEAS

BLACKBERRY MINT ICED TEA

MAKES ABOUT 8 1-CUP SERVINGS

This lovely recipe is not anything like the overly-sweet commercial iced teas on the market. It has only a hint of sweetness, making it very refreshing. It's also loaded with antioxidants thanks to the tea and berries. Add a squeeze of lemon or lime if it calls to you.

5   cups (1.25 L) water

5   black tea bags (Substitute white or green tea if desired.)

¼   cup (5 g) mint leaves, coarsely chopped

¼   cup (35 g) coconut sugar or other sweetener

6   cups (865 g) fresh or frozen blackberries

1. Bring the water to a boil in a large saucepot over high heat. Remove from the heat and add the tea bags and mint. Steep at least ten minutes.

2. Strain into a pitcher, discarding the tea bags and mint.

3. Stir in the sweetener.

4. Puree the blackberries in a blender or food processor; strain through a fine sieve if desired and discard the pulp.

5. Stir the blackberry puree into tea. Taste and adjust sugar as desired. Chill.

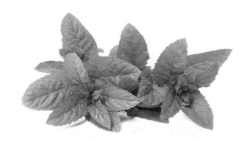

À VOTRE SANTÉ!

Here's something to consider about the antioxidant power of berries: In 2003, researchers from Azienda Policlinico Universitaria in Messina, Italy, observed that blackberry juice helped repair vascular tissue damaged by free radicals. What is in blackberries that enables them to fight free radicals? It is the compounds called anthocyanins, the very compounds that give blackberries their deep color.

BERRY ICED TEA

MAKES 7 1-CUP SERVINGS

This cool, berry-infused tea can be made with any kind of berry you have on hand—even a mix! It's a yummy, more health-supportive choice than store-bought iced tea drinks, which are loaded with sweeteners (often in the form of high-fructose corn syrup). For those of you who are making this for kids, or trying to lower the amount of caffeine you consume, see the option to make this with herbal tea.

> 1½ cups (185 g) fresh or frozen berries (raspberries, blackberries, blueberries, black currants, etc.)
>
> ¾ cup (175 ml) water
>
> ⅓ cup (50 g) coconut sugar or other natural sweetener
>
> 6 cups (1.5 L) hot brewed black tea or berry-flavored herbal tea (tea bags removed)

1. In a large saucepot over medium heat, simmer the berries, water, and coconut sugar until sugar dissolves and berries break apart.

2. Turn off the heat and add the hot tea. Allow to cool.

3. Strain the cooled liquid through a cheesecloth-lined sieve, pressing only lightly on the solids to keep the liquid clear. (For a thicker drink, feel free to puree the liquid, plus solids, in a high-powered blender.)

4. Chill until ready to enjoy.

BERRY-INFUSED ICED GREEN TEA

MAKES 4 1-CUP SERVINGS

Green tea is a darling of the health food world, said to help treat everything from headaches to obesity to Alzheimer's disease. Studies have shown that it does help prevent cardiovascular disease. And I happen to know it tastes great in this fruity berry tea!

> 4 cups (1 L) water
>
> ½ cup (60 g) raspberries
>
> ½ cup (60 g) strawberries, roughly chopped
>
> 4 bags green tea
>
> 2 teaspoons honey

1. In a saucepot over medium heat, bring the water to boil. Remove from the heat and add the tea bags, berries, and honey. Allow the mixture to steep for ten minutes.

2. Remove the tea bags and crush the berries with a potato masher or the back of a fork.

3. Strain the liquid through a sieve or colander, decanting into a pitcher.

4. Chill until cool.

MOCKTAILS

WATERMELON STRAWBERRY SIPPER

MAKES 2 1-CUP SERVINGS

What would summer be without one watermelon-based drink? Rich in lycopene (an antioxidant that helps strengthen the immune system and has been shown to prevent cancer), watermelon is a nutritious counterpart to the sprightly strawberry.

- 4   cups (620 g) cubed watermelon
- 1   cup (145 g) hulled strawberries
- 1   cup (250 ml) water
- 2   tablespoons lime juice
- 2   mint leaves

1. Add the watermelon, strawberries, water, lime juice, and mint leaves to a blender. Process until smooth. Thin with cold water if a thinner drink is desired.

2. Chill if desired before serving.

BRIGHT & BUBBLY

MAKES 2 1-CUP SERVINGS

This is a flexible recipe that lets you use whatever berries you have in your garden, fridge, or freezer.

- 2   cups (290 g) fresh or frozen berries of your choice (or a blend)
- 1   tablespoon lemon juice
- 2   tablespoons unfiltered honey
- 3   cups (700 ml) sparkling water

1. Add the berries, lemon juice, and honey to a blender and combine until smooth.

2. Scrape the puree into a pitcher, and when you are ready to serve, add the sparkling water, stirring gently until ingredients are combined.

LINGONBERRIES: DID YOU KNOW?

- It is said that lingonberries are sweeter when picked after a frost.
- Lingonberry leaves are rich in arbutin, a phytochemical that is used in whitening and brightening skincare products.
- Lingonberries' waxy leaves help the plant retain moisture.

SPARKLING RASPBERRY LIMEADE

MAKES 6 1-CUP SERVINGS

Homemade berry limeade is a very special drink. Plus, generous amounts of vitamin C make this a healthful nonalcoholic option. For something different, try this with lemons and strawberries or blackberries.

⅔ *cup (160 ml) lime juice*

½ *cup (125 ml) honey or (100 g) coconut sugar or raw cane sugar (Or yes, you can also use the same measure of table sugar.)*

1½ *cups (185 g) fresh or frozen (unsweetened thawed) raspberries*

3 *cups (700 ml) sparkling water*

1. Combine the lime juice and sweetener in a large pitcher, stirring to help dissolve the sweetener.

2. Place the berries in a fine-mesh sieve over a bowl. Use a rubber spatula to press on the berries, extracting the juice and some pulp while leaving the seeds behind. Stir the puree into the pitcher.

3. Just before serving, stir in the sparkling water. Serve over ice.

CRANBERRY FIZZ

MAKES 2 1-CUP SERVINGS

Sometimes you want a refreshing drink fast. Fiddling with whole berries can take work. For those times when you want a dressy, delicious, health-supportive, nonalcoholic drink, there's Cranberry Fizz!

1 *cup (250 ml) unsweetened cranberry juice (You can use any unsweetened berry juice here as well as unsweetened cherry or pomegranate juice.)*

1 *cup (250 ml) orange juice*

1 *cup (250 ml) sparkling water*

1. Add the cranberry and orange juices to a pitcher and stir.

2. Just before serving, stir in sparkling water. Serve over ice.

UTI BE GONE!

Several clinical studies have shown that drinking 8 to 10 ounces of cranberry juice daily may prevent half of all recurring urinary tract infections, according to a review in the June 2012 issue of *Clinics*. Researchers from Worcester Polytechnic Institute in Massachusetts found that the juice works by preventing E.coli bacteria from colonizing in the urinary tract.

COCKTAILS

BLUEBERRY BELLINI

MAKES 4 1-CUP SERVINGS

This is a quick, juice-based wine cocktail that is elegant and delicious and has the health benefits of blueberry juice, which is said to help strengthen eyesight and the immune system, help memory, and prevent cancer. Feel free to experiment with other juices.

1 *tablespoon unfiltered honey*

Juice of ½ lemon

2 *cups (475 ml) unsweetened blueberry juice*

2 *cups (475 ml) sparkling wine (such as Prosecco), divided*

1. In a blender, pulse together the honey, lemon juice, and blueberry juice.

2. Divide mixture among four champagne flutes. Top each with ½ cup sparkling wine.

BLUEBERRY JUICE
HELPS MAINTAIN MEMORY

More than one in every three people over the age of seventy in the United States have some form of memory loss. This number comes from a national study published in the November 2007 issue of *Neuroepidemiology* and conducted by a team of researchers at Duke University Medical Center, the University of Michigan, the University of Iowa, the University of Southern California, and the RAND Corporation. According to another study performed by a team at the University of Cincinnati and published in the January 2010 issue of *Journal of Agricultural and Food Chemistry*, blueberry juice may help many of these people.

Nine older adults with early memory changes were given between 6 and 9 ml of blueberry juice a day (depending upon their weight). At twelve weeks, researchers noted improved ability to learn new tasks and recall word lists. In addition, a reduction in symptoms of depression and lowered blood glucose levels occurred. If you or someone you know suffers from memory loss, enjoying a daily glass of blueberry juice could be worth a try.

BERRY SANGRIA

MAKES 6 1-CUP SERVINGS

Most sangria recipes call for some kind of sweetener. This one uses berries, wine, and seltzer. That is it. You'll love its fresh taste.

- 1   750-ml bottle chilled dry rosé wine *(Emphasis on the word dry; you don't want a sweet rosé.)*
- 1   *cup (250 ml) unsweetened cranberry juice or another unsweetened berry juice*
- 1   *cup (150 g) blueberries*
- 1   *cup (165 g) sliced strawberries*
- 1   *cup (145 g) blackberries or raspberries*
- 1   *cup (250 ml) chilled sparkling water*
- *Ice*

1. Combine the wine, juice, blueberries, strawberries, blackberries, and sparkling water in a large pitcher. Chill about four hours.

2. Just before serving, stir in sparkling water. Serve over ice.

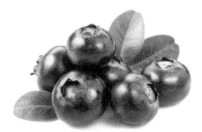

SCANDINAVIAN SPRITZER

MAKES 9 1-CUP SERVINGS

Although I grew up in Australia and the United States, my family is Danish. Thus, I have a soft spot for aquavit, the slightly spicy Danish spirit made from potatoes. Lingonberries are a northern European delicacy, prized for their benzoic acid, vitamins A and C, and magnesium. This recipe features both. You can use blueberries or cranberries (cousins of the lingonberry) if you want to change things up.

- 1   *tablespoon unfiltered honey or raw sugar*
- 1   *cup (250 ml) room-temperature water*
- ¾   *cup (75 g) fresh or frozen lingonberries*
- 4   *cups (1 L) soda water*
- 4   *cups (1 L) aquavit or vodka*
- *Ice*

1. Combine the honey and water in a blender. Pulse to dissolve the honey.

2. Add the lingonberries and pulse until completely blended.

3. Optional: Press the berry mixture through a sieve if a smooth drink is desired.

4. Pour the berry mixture into a large pitcher. Gently stir in the soda water and aquavit.

5. To serve, add ice to glasses before filling.

BERRY MELON SPARKLER

MAKES 2 1-CUP SERVINGS

Ah, Midori. . . . I probably shouldn't have this recipe in a health-related book on superfoods, but I have such fond memories of the various Midori-based drinks my friends and I used to concoct back in the day. Anyway, this one does have redeeming blackberries, which contain fiber and a host of antioxidants.

½ *cup (70 g) blackberries, plus a few more for garnish*

¼ *cup (60 ml) lemon juice*

½ *cup (125 ml) Midori liquor*

4 *ice cubes*

½ *cup (125 ml) Prosecco*

1. Muddle the berries and lemon juice in a cocktail shaker.

2. Add the Midori and ice cubes and shake vigorously.

3. Pour into wine glasses. Top with Prosecco, stir, and garnish with a few berries.

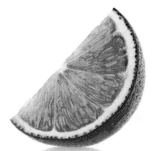

STRAWBERRY-ROSÉ SPRITZER

MAKES 8 1-CUP SERVINGS

This sparkling punch elevates any gathering. Plus, the strawberries are good for you!

1 *pint (290 g) strawberries, hulled and sliced*

1 *750-ml bottle rosé wine*

⅓ *cup unsweetened lingonberry, cherry, cranberry, pomegranate, or other red-colored fruit juice*

2 *cups (475 ml) sparkling water*

2 *tablespoons lemon juice*

1. Combine the strawberries and wine in a large pitcher; cover and chill for three hours.

2. Using a slotted spoon, remove the strawberries and set aside.

3. Stir the berry juice, sparkling water, and lemon juice into the pitcher of wine.

4. Remove 1 cup of the wine mixture from the pitcher, and add it to a blender with the reserved strawberries. Blend wine and strawberries until thoroughly liquefied.

5. Add wine-strawberry puree back to the pitcher, straining first through cheesecloth or a sieve if desired, to catch the remaining strawberry seeds.

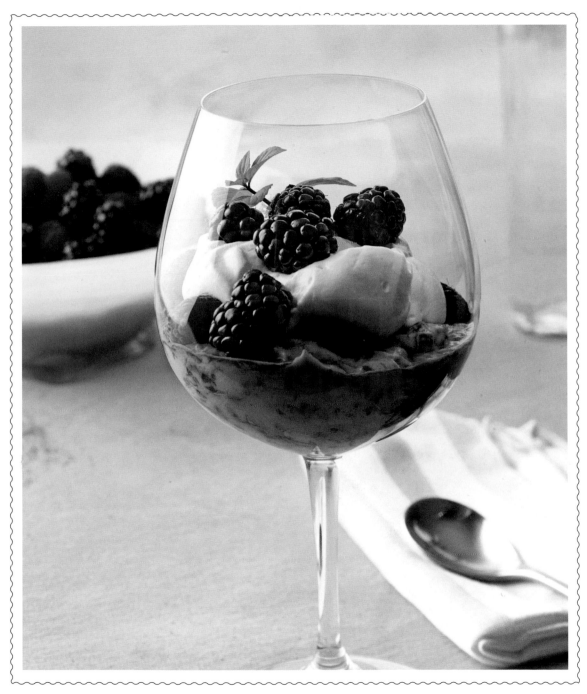

Berry Crème Parfait, page 144

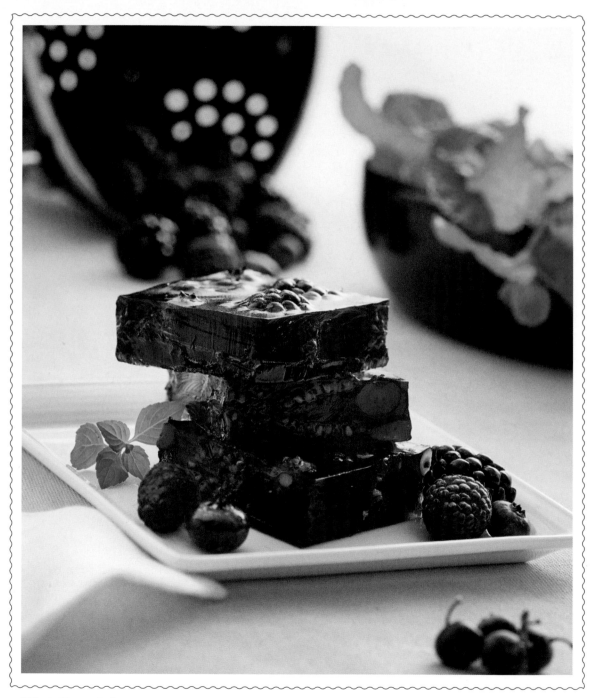

Whole Berry Gelatin, page 114

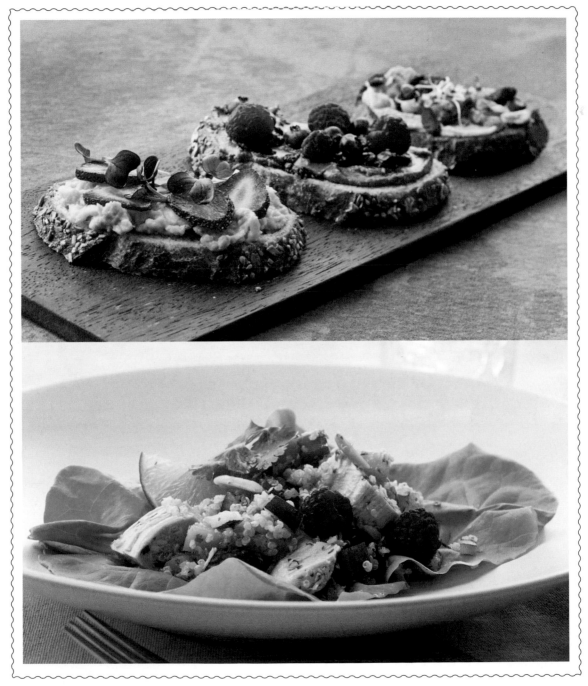

TOP: Avocado-Bean-Berry Sandwich and Berry Sandwich Ideas, pages 104 and 105
BOTTOM: Berry Main-Dish Salad Blueprint, page 119

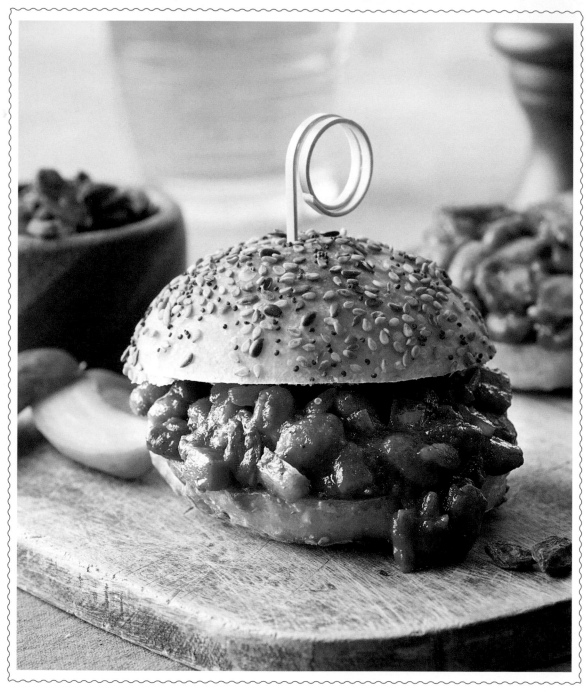

Slow Cooker Berry-Bean Sloppy Joes, page 124

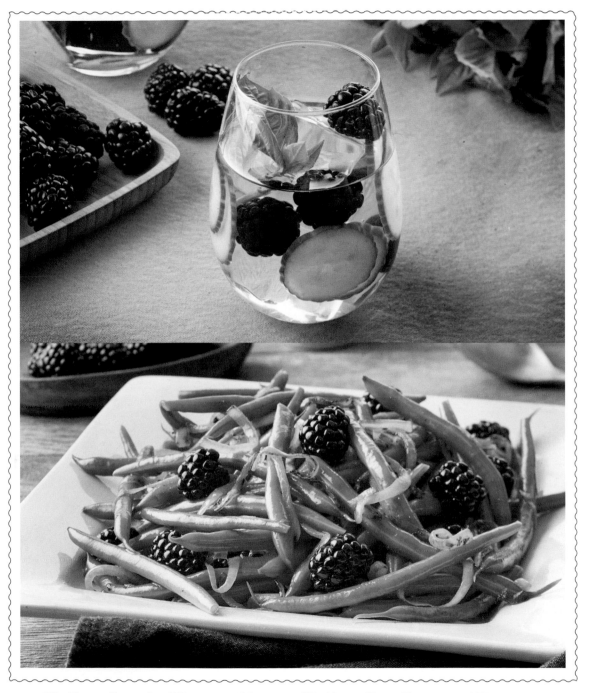

TOP: Blackberry Cucumber Water, page 55 BOTTOM: Blackberry Green Beans, page 137

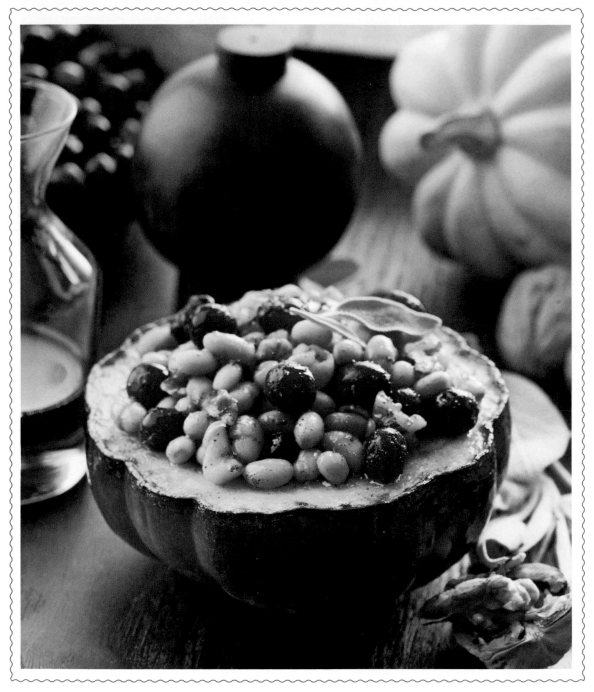

Acorn Squash with Walnuts & Cranberries, page 126

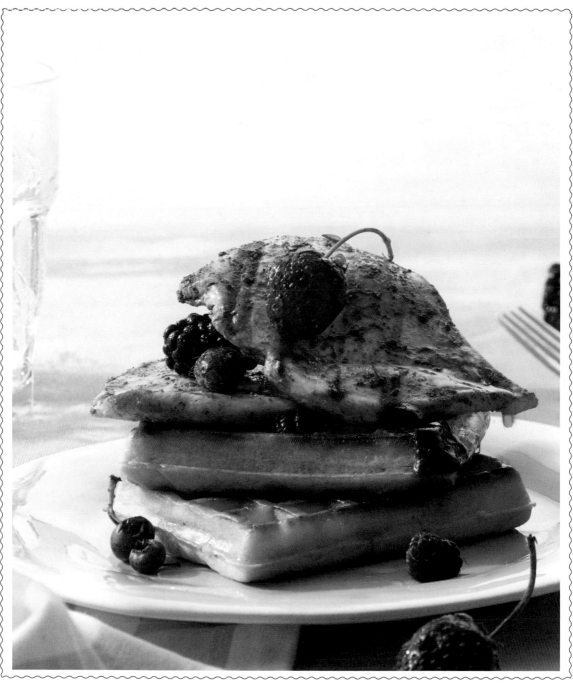

Gluten-Free Coconut-Berry Waffles (here topped with chicken breast and berry syrup), page 77

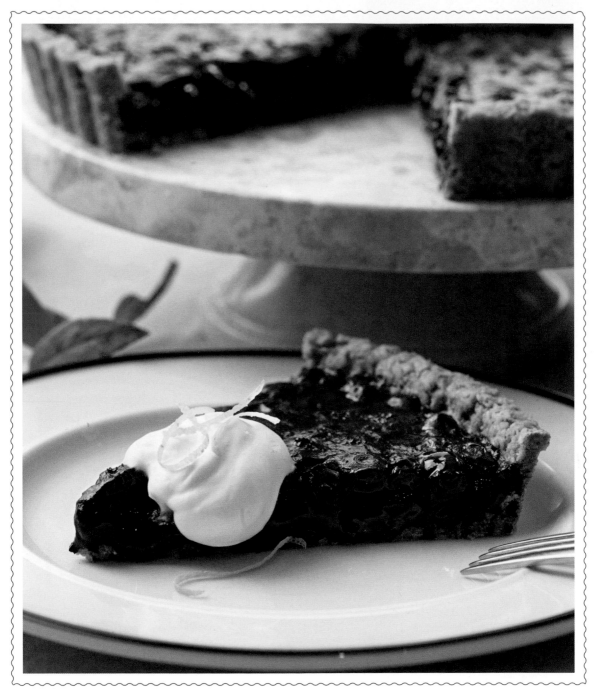

Blueberry Tart, page 152, with Whipped Coconut Cream, page 150

MEASUREMENT REMINDERS

- One pint of blueberries equals about 2½ cups (370 g) or ¾ pound of berries.

- One quart of blueberries equals about 4 cups (580 g) or 1½ pounds of berries.

- One 10-ounce (285 g) package frozen blueberries equals about 1½ cups (375 ml) of blueberries.

- One pint of strawberries equals 2 cups (500 ml) or ¾ pound (370 g) of sliced strawberries.

- One quart of strawberries equals about 4 cups (1 L) or 1½ pounds (600 g) of sliced strawberries.

- One 10-ounce (285 g) bag of frozen strawberries equals about 1½ cups (375 ml) of strawberries.

- One 6-ounce (170 g) package of fresh raspberries or blackberries equals about 1 cup (250 ml) and 1⅓ cups (334 ml), respectively, of berries, depending upon size of berries.

- One 16-ounce (426 g) carton of raspberries or blackberries equals about 3 cups (750 ml) and 4 cups (1 L), respectively of berries, depending upon size of berries.

- One pint of blackberries or raspberries equals about 1 cup (250 ml) to 1⅓ cups (334 ml) of berries, depending upon size of berries.

- One 10-ounce (285 g) bag of frozen raspberries or blackberries equals about 1¼ cups (265 ml) of berries, depending upon size of berries.

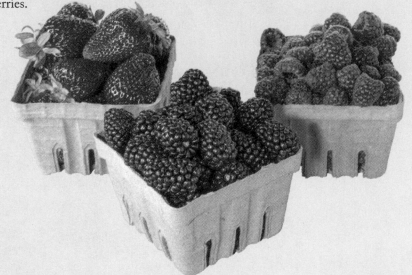

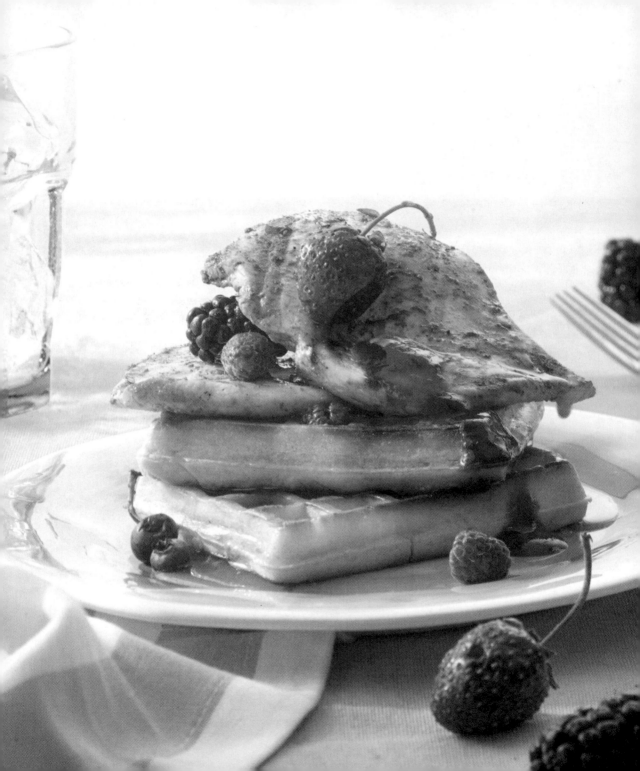

CHAPTER 4

BERRIES FOR BREAKFAST

Berries are a natural part of a morning meal. Traditionally, people enjoy berries stirred into yogurt, strewn atop a bowl of cold or hot cereal, tucked into a pancake or muffin, or made into a jam or fruit salad. And while these are all good ways to enjoy berries, I encourage you to expand your morning berry repertoire to include the new-fangled recipes in this chapter. They make the most of berries' great flavor and generous nutritional benefits.

MORNING BREADS & CAKES

BLUEBERRY BANANA OATMEAL BREAD

MAKES ABOUT 8 SERVINGS

Banana bread is a natural breakfast food, and it can be made even healthier with fiber-rich oats, nourishing applesauce, protein-packed nuts, and antioxidant-heavy berries.

1 cup (80 g) quick or old-fashioned oats

1½ (85 g) cups spelt flour

⅓ cup (50 g) brown sugar

1 teaspoon baking soda

½ teaspoon salt

Optional: 1 teaspoon ground cinnamon or ginger or a combination

2 eggs

1 teaspoon vanilla extract

½ cup (125 ml) unsweetened applesauce or pumpkin puree

2 large bananas, peeled and mashed

½ cup (50 g) pecans or walnuts, chopped

1 cup (150 g) blueberries

1. Preheat oven to 350°F (175°C or gas mark 4). Grease a loaf pan.

2. In a medium bowl, whisk together the oats, spelt flour, brown sugar, baking soda, salt, and cinnamon.

3. In a separate bowl, whisk together the eggs, vanilla extract, and applesauce until well blended. Stir in the mashed bananas.

(continued)

OPPOSITE: Gluten-Free Coconut-Berry Waffles, page 77

4. Pour the liquid mixture into the dry mixture and stir together. Carefully fold in the nuts and the blueberries.

5. Pour the batter into the loaf pan and bake for 1 hour or until bread is springy to the touch.

6. Allow to cool in the pan before removing. Wrap uneaten bread in food wrap and store for up to three days at room temperature. Or wrap and freeze for up to three months.

GLUTEN-FREE BLUEBERRY CORN MUFFINS

MAKES 10 TO 12 SERVINGS

Some of us have loved ones who either cannot or don't want to eat gluten. This is why it's important to have some good gluten-free recipes in your repertoire. This muffin recipe is a variation on one that I made for my oldest son when he was a toddler and on a strict gluten-free diet to heal his leaky gut, a condition where small perforations occur in the large instestines. Undigested food can pass through these tears and into the bloodstream.

- 1¼ cups (200 g) finely ground yellow cornmeal
- 1 scant cup (125 g) gluten-free all-purpose flour blend
- 1 teaspoon baking powder
- 1 teaspoon baking soda
- ¼ teaspoon salt
- ½ cup (125 ml) liquid coconut oil
- ½ cup (125 ml) coconut milk (do not use light)
- ¼ cup (60 ml) Grade B maple syrup
- 4 large eggs
- 1 cup (150 g) fresh or unthawed frozen blueberries, blackberries, or raspberries

1. Preheat oven to 400°F (205°C or gas mark 6).

2. Prepare a muffin tin by lining with paper cups.

3. In large bowl, whisk together the cornmeal, gluten-free flour, baking powder, baking soda, and salt.

4. In another large bowl, whisk together the coconut oil, coconut milk, maple syrup, and eggs.

5. Pour the wet ingredients into the dry ingredients and stir until fully combined.

6. Gently fold in the berries.

7. Distribute the batter among muffin cups, filling each cup three-quarters full. Bake until tops are domed and feel springy to the touch, and a toothpick inserted in the center comes out clean, about fifteen minutes. Let cool in the pan five minutes, then turn out onto a wire rack.

PALEO-STYLE STRAWBERRY PANCAKES

MAKES 4 SERVINGS

In this yummy gluten-free pancake recipe, coconut—in the forms of flour, oil, nectar, and milk—plays a starring role. Coconut boasts powerful antimicrobial properties, strengthens the immune system, and supports heart and brain health. Here, its rich, tropical taste pairs beautifully with sweet, vitamin-rich strawberries. These pancakes cook most thoroughly and are easiest to flip when made "Swedish style," or in other words, on the small side.

- ½ cup (56 g) coconut flour
- ½ teaspoon baking powder
- ¼ teaspoon salt
- 6 eggs, at room temperature
- ¼ cup (50 ml) liquid coconut oil, plus more for the skillet
- 1 tablespoon coconut nectar
- 1 cup (250 ml) coconut milk
- 1 cup (200 g) chopped strawberries

1. In a large bowl, whisk together the coconut flour, baking powder, and salt until combined.

2. In another large bowl, whisk together the eggs, coconut oil, coconut nectar, and coconut milk.

3. Pour the dry ingredients into the wet ingredients and stir until just blended.

4. Gently fold in the strawberries.

5. Brush a skillet with a bit of coconut oil and place over medium-low heat.

6. For each pancake, ladle a few tablespoons of pancake batter onto the hot skillet and cook until golden. Flip and cook remaining side until golden.

GLUTEN-FREE COCONUT-BERRY WAFFLES

MAKES 4 SERVINGS

Although I won't deny eating gluten-containing foods once in awhile, I feel so much better without gluten in my body. That's why I always include gluten-free recipes in my cookbooks. If you haven't yet tried adding gluten-free options to some of your favorite breakfast foods, try waffles. Unlike gluten-free bread, cakes, and cookies—which many people find dry or gummy—almost everyone loves gluten-free pancakes and waffles. This hearty waffle boasts protein from nuts, lauric acid from coconut, and nourishing berries.

- 3 tablespoons coconut flour
- ¼ teaspoon salt

(continued)

¾ teaspoon baking soda

Optional: Dash of ground cinnamon

3 eggs

1 cup (145 g) raw almonds or cashews

⅓ cup (80 ml) coconut milk

3 tablespoons coconut nectar, honey, or Grade B maple syrup

3 tablespoons liquid coconut oil

1. Preheat your waffle iron and oil it if required.

2. In a large bowl, whisk together the coconut flour, salt, baking soda, and optional cinnamon. Set aside.

3. In a food processor, add the eggs, nuts, coconut milk, coconut nectar, and coconut oil. Process until mixture is smooth.

4. Add the coconut flour mixture to the food processor and pulse just to blend.

5. Pour the batter into the waffle iron, being careful not to overfill. These waffles do rise, so you want the batter to barely cover the iron.

6. Cook the waffles for about a minute or until they are lightly golden and release easily with a fork when the lid is opened.

7. Repeat with the remaining batter.

MAKE YOUR OWN BERRY BREAKFAST SYRUP

MAKES ABOUT 1¾ CUPS (425 ML)

Breakfast syrup is a great place to sneak more fruit into your diet. This yummy syrup is super easy and super customizable. Just substitute any berry for the blackberries. I've made this syrup with mulberries, black currants, lingonberries, raspberries, blueberries, and strawberries—and they've all been great.

3 cups (432 g) fresh or frozen (no need to thaw) blackberries

1 tablespoon Grade D maple syrup, coconut nectar, honey, or another sweetener

¼ cup (50 ml) water

1. Add the berries, sweetener, and water to a medium saucepot over medium-high heat and simmer for five minutes.

2. Transfer the mixture to a food processor or blender and process until completely smooth.

3. Return the mixture to the saucepot and allow it to simmer over medium heat until the syrup has slightly reduced and become as thick as honey.

CEREALS

NUTS & SEEDS GRANOLA

MAKES 3 CUPS (350 G)

This is my go-to granola—I've been making it for years. Go ahead and personalize it by using whatever nut or seed butter you'd like, try a different liquid sweetener, and play with other nuts and dried fruits.

- 4   tablespoons peanut butter
- 4   tablespoons honey
- ½   teaspoon ground cinnamon
- ½   teaspoon vanilla extract
- 2   cups (160 g) old-fashioned oats
- ½   cup chopped nuts of choice (or use sunflower or pumpkin seeds)
- ½   cup dried goji berries or dried unsweetened cranberries

1. Preheat oven to 325°F (160°C or gas mark 3).

2. Line a baking sheet with parchment paper or a baking mat.

3. In a large bowl, combine the nut butter and honey and microwave until the nut butter and honey have melted. Or melt in a large saucepot over low heat. Stir together and then add the cinnamon and vanilla.

4. Add the oats and nuts and stir until all the oats are coated with the mixture.

5. Spread the mixture in a single layer on the baking sheet and bake for about fourteen minutes or until the granola is golden, fragrant, and almost dry. (Granola continues to firm up when removed from the oven, so do not overbake it.)

6. Remove from oven and let cool completely on the sheet. Mix in dried berries.

7. Store in an airtight container for up to two weeks.

THE MIGHTY OAT

Rolled oats come from the grain of the oat plant. After harvesting, oats are minimally processed—the manufactuer removes the hull of the oat grain and grinds the grain into coarse flakes. A one-cup (150 g) serving of cooked rolled oats—aka oatmeal—contains about 166 calories and boasts 4 g of dietary fiber and 5.9 g of protein, as well as thiamine, phosphorus, magnesium, iron, and copper.

NUT-FREE HIGH PROTEIN GRANOLA

MAKES 8 SERVINGS

For those of you don't like nuts or can't eat them, there is another way to infuse your granola with extra protein: protein powder.

- 3 cups (450 g) old-fashioned oats
- ½ teaspoon ground cinnamon
- ½ teaspoon ground allspice
- ½ cup (120 ml) unsweetened apple or pear juice
- ⅓ cup (80 ml) Grade B maple syrup
- ⅔ cup (65 g) brown rice protein powder
- 3 tablespoons liquid coconut oil
- ¼ teaspoon salt
- 2 teaspoons vanilla extract
- ¼ cup (25 g) dried goji berries
- ½ cup (60 g) dried unsweetened cranberries (or another dried or freeze-dried berry)

1. Preheat oven to 325°F (160°C or gas mark 3).

2. Line a large baking sheet with parchment paper or a baking mat.

3. In a large bowl, combine the oats, cinnamon, and allspice. Set aside.

4. In a medium saucepot over medium heat, whisk together the apple or pear juice, maple syrup, protein powder, coconut oil, and salt, until the mixture is smooth and thick.

5. When the mixture begins to bubble, whisk in vanilla.

6. Pour the liquid mixture over the oats mixture, stirring to combine

7. Spread the mixture in a single layer onto prepared baking sheet, being careful not to crowd the ingredients.

8. Bake in preheated oven for forty to forty-five minutes, stirring once or twice, or until granola is golden, fragrant, and almost dry. (Granola continues to firm up when removed from the oven, so do not overbake it.)

9. Remove from the oven and let cool completely on the sheet. Once cool, stir in the goji berries and cranberries.

10. Store in an airtight container for up to two weeks.

GOJI BERRIES FOR VIRILITY

In ancient China, goji berries were a popular male libido and virility enhancer. They were so powerful, it was thought, that men were advised not to consume them while away from their family, for fear of what they may do. As the old Chinese saying goes, "A man who is leaving on a long way far from home should not take goji with him."

GRANOLA COOKIES

MAKES 12 SERVINGS

Cookies for breakfast? Well . . . I have to admit, I probably wouldn't serve these for breakfast every day (I like my clients to have green drinks and protein for breakfast), but they are fantastic for brunch or for the kids (who have faster metabolisms than we adults) to grab-and-go as they rush to school, rehearsals, or practice.

1   cup (150 g) pitted Medjool dates

1   large ripe banana, peeled

¾   cup (175 ml) unsweetened applesauce

¼   cup (50 ml) coconut oil, melted

1   tablespoon coconut nectar (or agave nectar)

2   cups (300 g) blueberries (or dried
     unsweetened) or cranberries

2½ cups (200 g) old-fashioned oats

1   cup (220 g) unsweetened coconut flakes

5   tablespoons chia seeds

½   cup (60 g) chopped walnuts, almonds,
     cashews, pecans, or other nuts

½   cup (70 g) sunflower seeds

½   teaspoon ground cinnamon

½   teaspoon ground allspice

½   teaspoon salt

1. Preheat oven to 350°F (175°C or gas mark 4).

2. Line a baking sheet with parchment paper or foil.

3. Place the dates and banana in a food processor and pulse until the dates are very finely diced.

4. In a large bowl, stir together the date mixture, applesauce, coconut oil, and coconut nectar until well combined.

5. Add the blueberries and gently stir.

6. In a separate bowl, whisk together the oats, coconut, chia, nuts, sunflower seeds, cinnamon, allspice, and salt.

7. Add the dry ingredients to the fruit mixture and stir until thoroughly combined.

8. Using a tablespoon or small cookie scoop, place balls of the batter onto the prepared cookie sheet. Using wet fingertips or the bottom of a glass tumbler, flatten the cookies to half-inch thick.

9. Bake for thirty minutes, until they are fragrant and the bottom of the cookies are golden. Allow cookies to cool on the baking sheet. Though they may seem a bit soft when you remove them from the oven, they will firm up as they cool on the baking sheet.

10. Transfer them to an airtight container and store for up to five days.

BERRY BREAKFAST POLENTA

MAKES 4 SERVINGS

Jamaica's turned cornmeal, America's Indian pudding, Italy's polenta—dried corn is a versatile food that can create a filling, delicious breakfast. Don't believe me? Try this Berry Breakfast Polenta! (*Note:* This recipe calls for a mix of berries, but please feel free to stick to one type if you'd like. You'll still get delicious results.)

FOR THE BERRY SAUCE

- 1   *tablespoon liquid coconut oil*
- 3   *tablespoons coconut nectar or coconut sugar*
- 1   *tablespoon lemon juice*
- 1   *12-ounce (340 g) bag assorted frozen berries (Fresh is fine too.)*

FOR THE POLENTA

- 3   *cups (770 ml) coconut milk*
- ½   *cup (80 g) instant polenta*
- 2   *tablespoons coconut sugar*
- ½   *teaspoon salt*

1. Add coconut oil to a medium saucepot over medium heat. Add the coconut nectar, lemon juice, and berries. Whisk to combine.

2. Bring the mixture to a boil and reduce heat to medium-low. Simmer for about five minutes, or until the mixture is slightly reduced and the berries have softened.

3. Add the coconut milk to a medium saucepot over medium heat. Bring to a boil.

4. Slowly add the polenta, a bit at a time, stirring constantly with a whisk.

5. After all the polenta has been added, stir in the coconut sugar and salt. Continue stirring constantly until the mixture is thick. Remove from the heat and set aside.

6. Ladle the polenta into four shallow bowls and top with the berry sauce.

THE HISTORY OF POLENTA

Once upon a time, polenta—known in the days of ancient Rome as *pulmentum*—was a humble, everyday grain mush (think porridge) eaten by everyone and made from a variety of startchy ingredients, including farro, chestnut flour, millet, spelt, and ground chickpeas. Corn became the official ingredient of polenta as we know it today when explorers brought it to Europe, from the Americas, in sixteenth century.

- The blackberry is the state fruit of both Kentucky and Alabama.

- Blackberry bushes, thanks to their vicious thorns, were often planted around European villages to offer protection against enemies and large animals that might do harm.

- Tea made from blackberry leaves is a traditional cure for diarrhea and dysentery. It is believed that the high level of astringent tannins in the leaves helps the body absorb excess liquid in the digestive tract.

- The astringency in blackberry leaves also helps clean wounds, while encouraging blood vessels to constrict and bleeding to stop. The astringent qualities of blackberry leaves may also prove useful in soothing a sore throat and treating hemorrhoids.

BERRY BREAKFAST QUINOA

MAKES 2 SERVINGS

When my boys were babies, breakfast quinoa was the first quinoa dish they ate. Soothing, delicious, and deeply nourishing, this recipe leaves you feeling both satisfied and energized. Dress it with coconut milk and blueberries or another berry of your choice.

1   *tablespoon liquid coconut oil*

½   *cup (85 g) dry quinoa, rinsed and patted dry*

¾   *cup (175 ml) coconut milk*

1   *teaspoon vanilla extract*

Pinch of salt

¼   *teaspoon ground ginger*

¼   *teaspoon ground cinnamon*

½   *cup (75 g) blueberries*

Squirt of lemon juice

Optional: Splash of milk, sweetener of your choice, and chopped nuts

1. Add the coconut oil and quinoa to a small saucepot over medium heat. Toast for two or so minutes, or until fragrant.

2. Add the coconut milk, vanilla, salt, ginger, and cinnamon and bring to a boil. Immediately reduce the heat to very low, toss in the blueberries (no need to stir), cover the pan, and simmer mixture for fifteen minutes or until quinoa is tender and the liquid has cooked away.

3. Fluff the quinoa with a fork and divide into two bowls. Enjoy as-is or with an optional splash of coconut milk, sweetener of choice, and a sprinkle of chopped nuts.

BAKED BERRY OATMEAL

MAKES 6 SERVINGS

Baked oatmeal is a delicious take on bread pudding: It is hearty, fiber-filled, and easily dressed with fresh, frozen, or dried fruit (berries in this case). Because it's hearty and forgiving (as well as delicious), it makes a great make-ahead brunch or weekend dish.

2   cups (160g) rolled oats

1   cup (50 g) walnuts or pecans, chopped, divided

1   teaspoon baking powder

Pinch of salt

1   teaspoon ground cinnamon

½   teaspoon ground allspice

½   teaspoon salt

2   cups (475 ml) coconut milk

⅓   cup (80 ml) Grade B maple syrup

1   large egg

3   tablespoons liquid coconut oil, divided, plus
    a bit more to oil the baking pan

2   teaspoons vanilla extract

2   bananas, sliced into ½-inch (1.25 cm) pieces
    (Or use a chopped pear or chopped apple.)

1½ (150 g) cups cranberries, blueberries, or
    a mix of berries, divided (Or use leftover
    whole berry cranberry sauce.)

1. Preheat oven to 375°F (190°C or gas mark 5).

2. Oil the bottoms and sides of an 8-inch (20-cm) square baking pan. Set aside.

3. In a large bowl, whisk together the oats, ½ cup of the nuts, baking powder, salt, cinnamon, and allspice.

4. In another bowl, whisk together the coconut milk, maple syrup, egg, 1½ tablespoons of the coconut oil, and the vanilla.

5. Pour the liquid mixture over the oat mixture and stir until all ingredients are combined. Set aside.

6. Scatter the chopped bananas in a single layer across the bottom of prepared baking pan. Top the bananas with the berries.

7. Spoon the oat mixture over the bananas and berries, trying not to disturb them too much.

8. Scatter the remaining berries and ½ cup of nuts over the top.

9. Bake for forty to forty-five minutes, until the top is golden and the oats are set.

10. Drizzle with the remaining 1½ tablespoons coconut oil and cool for ten minutes before slicing and serving.

IN A JAM? TRY THIS!

MAKES ABOUT 1½ CUPS (350 ML)

If we're being honest about our health, we could probably do without the insane amount of sugar most jams contain. That's why I included a recipe for super-easy, fresh-tasting jam that contains coconut sugar, a mineral-rich, low-carboydrate sweetener that has a low glycemic index. You've got to try it!

- 1 *pound (450 g) fresh or thawed strawberries, quartered*
- 2 *tablespoons water*
- ⅔ *cup coconut sugar*
- 1 *large apple (any variety), peeled and coarsely grated*
- 1 *tablespoon lemon juice*

1. Combine the strawberries, water, and sugar in a large heavy skillet over medium-high heat. Heat the ingredients, stirring until coconut sugar begins to dissolve.

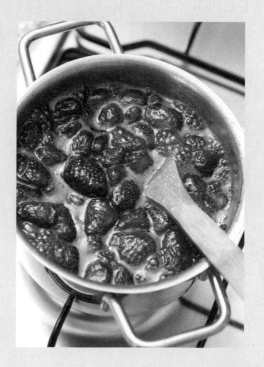

2. Stir in the grated apple. Cook the mixture over medium-low heat, stirring occasionally and breaking up the strawberries, until the sugar dissolves. With a potato masher or the back of a fork, gently smash the berries to desired texture.

3. Simmer the mixture until the jam is thickened, about ten to fifteen minutes. Stir in the lemon juice.

4. Let cool—the mixture will continue to thicken as it cools—and transfer to a tightly covered container. Refrigerate and use within two weeks.

ACAI BERRY BREAKFAST BOWL

MAKES 2 SERVINGS

I first heard of acai bowls from one of my clients, who was addicted to them. I pumped up her acai bowl with a bit of spinach and some protein and came up with this fruity version.

1   *fresh or frozen banana, peeled*

2   *cups (245 g) fresh or frozen berries (one type or a blend of berries)*

1   *small handful baby spinach*

2   *Medjool dates*

1   *tablespoon chia*

1   *tablespoon cashew or almond butter*

1   *heaping tablespoon acai powder*

Optional garnish: Chopped nuts or sunflower seeds

1. Place all the ingredients in a food processor and process until smooth.

2. Divide between two shallow bowls and garnish if desired with nuts or seeds.

STRAWBERRY CHIA PUDDING

MAKES 2 SERVINGS

If you have seen any of my other cookbooks, you'll know that I include a chia pudding recipe in all of them. This version is fruity and super yummy. You'll get protein, fiber, and a host of antioxidants too. Make it the night before you plan to eat it, and you'll have something delicious to wake up to!

18 *ounces (510 g) strawberries (Raspberries are also good.)*

2   *tablespoons coconut nectar*

4   *tablespoons chia seeds*

1. In a blender or food processor, process the strawberries and coconut nectar until smooth.

2. Add the chia seeds and pulse until smooth.

3. Scrape the mixture into a covered container and chill for three hours or more to thicken.

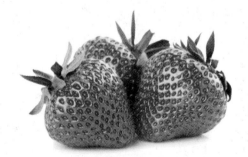

EGGS

BANANA BERRY OMELET

MAKES 1 LARGE OMELET OR 2 SMALL OMELETS

Here's another omelet that is full of berries. This one is made even sweeter with the addition of banana. Kids love this!

1   *medium to large banana*
2   *eggs*
Pinch of ground cinnamon
2   *teaspoons liquid coconut oil*
1   *cup (100 g) mixed berries*

1. Add the banana to a large bowl and, using the back of a fork, mash it into a paste.

2. Add the eggs and cinnamon to the banana and whisk until the ingredients are fully blended.

3. Add the coconut oil to a frying pan set over medium heat.

4. Add the egg mixture to the pan and cook for one to two minutes, until it begins to set.

5. Add berries and cook just until eggs are ready.

6. Remove the omelet from the pan by running a spatula under the edges and then sliding it onto a plate.

BERRY OMELET

MAKES 1 LARGE OMELET OR 2 SMALL OMELETS

When I first moved to New York City, one of the most intriguing things on Manhattan diner breakfast menus was a jelly omelet. This recipe is an homage to that old-time New York favorite.

1   *cup (100 g) blueberries*
1   *tablespoon water*
2   *eggs*
½   *teaspoon vanilla extract*
½   *teaspoon ground cinnamon*
1   *tablespoon coconut, almond, or other oil*

1. Add the blueberries and water to a small saucepot and cook over medium-high heat until the blueberries soften, five to ten minutes. Remove from the heat and set aside.

2. In a large bowl, whisk together the eggs, vanilla, and cinnamon.

3. Add the oil to a frying pan over medium heat. Pour in the egg mixture and cook until it sets.

4. Remove the omelet from the pan by running a spatula under the edges and then sliding it onto a plate.

5. Spoon the berry mixture over the omelet.

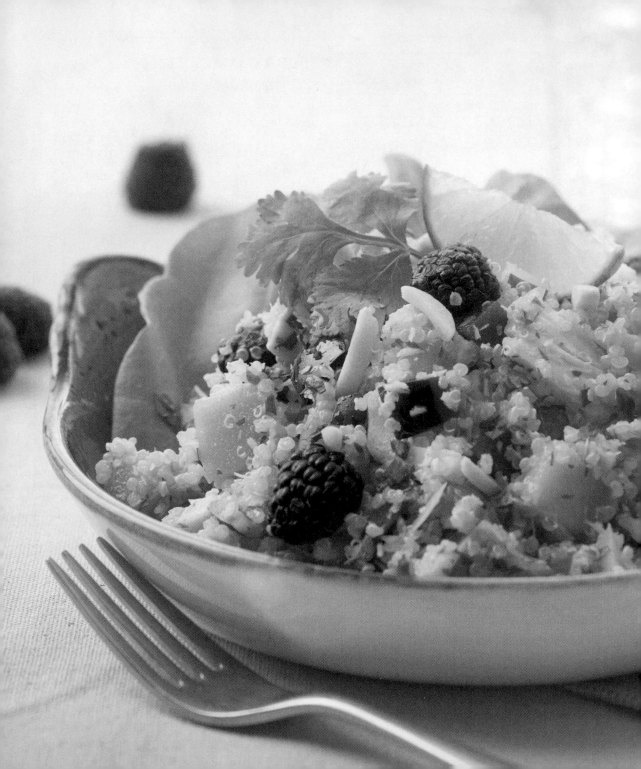

CHAPTER 5

BERRIES FOR LUNCH

I realize that berries are not traditionally thought of as a lunch food, but the combination of fiber, antioxidants, and flavor berries offer makes them the perfect addition to this important meal. You see, for me, lunch really is the most important meal of the day. Midday is when your body is busiest and needs the right fuel to power through a marathon of mental, physical, and emotional tasks.

But too many of us have a grab-and-go mentality when it comes to lunch—grab a sandwich, hamburger, or slice of pizza and go, go, go. The problem, however, with gulping down nutrient-poor food is it can make you feel sluggish, upset your stomach, and leave you feeling spacey and irritable. Worse yet, it puts you on a hamster wheel of cravings for more and more junky food, a track that makes it difficult to feel energized or productive.

The right lunch—one made with nutrient-dense superfoods, such as berries—can energize you and leave you feeling satisfied, intellectually sharp, happy, and powerful. Berries can help with that. Really. They contain energizing vitamin C, satisfying fiber, vitamin A to help with mental acuity, and so many more beneficial nutrients. For me, lunching on a berry-packed smoothie and a berry-quinoa bowl leaves me feeling vibrant, filled with vigor, and ready to address anything that comes my way.

Ready to get on top of your game? Enjoy a berry lunch and see how great you feel afterward!

CHILIS, STEWS & SOUPS

RASPBERRY BUFFALO SLOW COOKER CHILI

MAKES 10 SERVINGS

At first glance, berries and chili may not seem like the most simpatico of combinations. But keep an open mind! I assure you that the sweet-tart zingy taste of raspberries elevates

(continued)

OPPOSITE: **Quinoa Coconut Chicken Bowl, page 102**

chili to a gourmet experience (while adding more antioxidants and fiber to an already nutrient-packed food.) This recipe calls for raspberries, but I have used blueberries, red currants, and blackberries with good results. And if you don't like bison, go ahead and use hamburger, or even a mix of hamburger and ground pork. Or make it vegetarian by replacing the meat with five cans of your favorite beans. You'll need a 6-quart (6.5 L) slow cooker for this one, but you can also make it on the stovetop.

1   tablespoon extra-virgin olive oil

3   pounds (1.36 kg) ground bison

1   16-ounce (450 g) can black beans

3   14½-ounce (410 g) cans diced tomatoes

2   6-ounce (170 g) cans tomato paste

16 ounces (450 g) fresh or frozen raspberries

2   red, yellow, or orange bell peppers, diced

2   jalapeno or serrano chiles, deseeded and minced

2   zucchini or crookneck squashes, diced

1   small or medium onion, diced

3   cloves garlic, minced

1   tablespoon dried oregano

1   tablespoon cumin

1   teaspoon ground pepper

1   tablespoon mild chili powder

½   teaspoon salt

1. Add the olive oil to a slow cooker and distribute to evenly coat the bottom.

2. Add all the remaining ingredients, stirring to combine.

3. Turn the slow cooker to the low setting and cook for eight hours, stirring at least once during cooking if possible.

4. Adjust seasoning before serving.

CUMIN: IT'S GOOD FOR YOU!

Cumin is a popular ingredient in chili and Mexican-inspired dishes. Here's more information about this good-for-you spice:

The seed is a rich source of iron, a mineral that plays many vital roles in the body.

In some cultures, including the West Indies, India, Pakistan, and Mexico, cumin is used as a digestive aid. Recent research has indeed found that cumin stimulates the secretion of pancreatic enzymes, which help with digestion and nutrient assimilation.

Cumin boasts anti-carcinogenic properties. In one study, cumin was shown to protect laboratory animals from developing stomach or liver tumors.

High in antioxidants, cumin enhances the body's immune system function.

RED CURRANT COCOA STEW

MAKES 6 SERVINGS

Although most home cooks in the United States rarely combine beef and red currants, it's popular in England, and no wonder: the bright, tart flavor of fresh red currants adds an appealing freshness to beef dishes. Red currants also add vitamin C and immunity-strengthening phytonutrients to this protein-rich dish. To make it, you'll need a large pot that can go from stovetop to oven safely.

- 5 *tablespoons extra-virgin olive oil, divided*
- 1 *pound (450 g) stewing beef, preferably in 1½- to 2-inch (4-cm to 5-cm) cubes*
- 2 *shallots, minced*
- 2 *cloves garlic, minced*
- 2 *medium carrots, chopped*
- 2 *celery stalks, chopped*
- 1 *tablespoon finely chopped fresh rosemary*
- 3 *tablespoons all-purpose, whole-wheat, or gluten-free flour*
- 1 *tablespoon cocoa powder*
- 1 *cup (110 g) red currants*
- 1½ *cups (350 ml) cabernet wine*
- 3 *cups (700 ml) beef broth*

1. Preheat oven to 400°F (205°C or gas mark 6).

2. Add 2 tablespoons of the olive oil to a large ovenproof pot and place over high heat. Add the beef and quickly brown on all sides, being careful not to cook the beef through.

3. Turn the heat down to medium and add the shallots, garlic, carrots, celery, and rosemary and sauté for another two minutes.

4. Add the remaining 3 tablespoons of olive oil and the flour and cocoa powder and stir until dissolved.

5. Add the currants and wine. Simmer until the wine has reduced by half.

6. Add the broth and allow the stew to come to a simmer.

7. Immediately cover the stew pot, remove it from the heat, and carefully place it in the oven and bake for forty-five minutes.

8. Remove the pot from the oven, uncover it, and allow the stew to sit for fifteen minutes before serving.

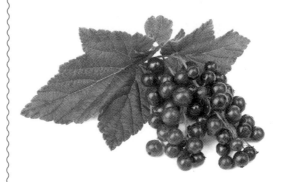

QUINOA CRANBERRY RED SOUP

MAKES 4 SERVINGS

Many vegetarian soups rely on beans for their protein. Not this interesting soup! Instead, it contains red quinoa, a terrific source of vegetarian protein, fiber, amino acids, iron, magnesium, and vitamin B_6. The cranberries add zing and phytonutrients. You'll need already-cooked quinoa for this one. If you don't have red quinoa, use the regular kind.

1   cup (100 g) cranberries
1   cup (30 g) spinach, chopped
1   cup (124 g) zucchini, diced
4   cups (1 L) vegetable broth
1   tablespoon liquid coconut oil
1   shallot, finely chopped
1   tablespoon lemon grass, chopped
1   cup (185 g) red quinoa, cooked
¼   cup (50 ml) unsweetened coconut milk
2   tablespoons fresh cilantro, chopped
Salt and pepper, to taste

1. In a large saucepot, combine the cranberries, spinach, zucchini, and vegetable broth.

2. Bring to a boil over medium-high heat.

3. Cover the pan and remove from the heat. Set aside.

4. In the meantime, heat the oil in another large saucepot over medium heat. Add the shallot and lemongrass and cook for two minutes or until fragrant.

5. Add the quinoa and sauté for a minute. Remove from the heat and set aside.

6. Pureé the cranberry-vegetable-broth mixture using a blender, handheld blender, or food processor until completely smooth.

7. Add the pureed cranberry broth to the quinoa mixture and cook over medium-high heat until it begins to simmer. Simmer for two minutes.

8. Add the coconut milk, cilantro, and salt and pepper and remove from the heat and serve.

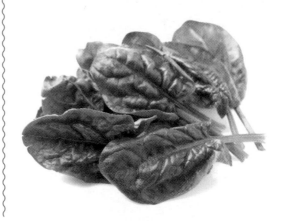

CUCUMBER & GOOSEBERRY SOUP

MAKES 4 SERVINGS

This is what my friends affectionately call a "lady soup"—a delicacy you can serve alongside tea sandwiches at an afternoon get-together. This soup is refreshing thanks to detoxifying cucumber, and features that British favorite, gooseberry. It is great warm, chilled, or at room temperature. Leave out the fish if you want a vegetarian soup.

1 tablespoon liquid coconut oil

1 small onion, chopped

3 to 4 hothouse cucumbers (or about 2 pounds [905 g] small cucumbers) seeded and sliced

1 cup (150 g) diced potato (about 1 large potato)

1 cup (150 g) gooseberries

1 cup (250 ml) chicken or vegetable broth

1 cup (250 ml) coconut cream (not cream of coconut)

Salt and pepper, to taste

½ cup (70 g) smoked salmon, cooked trout, or cooked shrimp, sliced or chopped

1. Add the coconut oil and onion to a large saucepot over medium heat. Cook until softened, about five minutes.

(continued)

2. Add the cucumber, potato, and gooseberries, and stir for a minute before adding the broth. Bring to a simmer, cover, and turn heat to low. Simmer twenty minutes or until the potatoes are tender, stirring periodically.

3. Allow the mixture to cool slightly before pouring it into a food processor or blender. Process until completely smooth.

4. Add the coconut cream to the mixture and process until combined. Season with salt and pepper.

5. Serve the soup at room temperature, or return it to the pan and warm it slightly or chill and serve cold.

6. To serve, ladle the soup into six bowls and top each bowl with some of the salmon, trout, or shrimp.

GOOSEBERRY FEVER

The early 1800s were a time of gooseberry mania. At the height of the berry's popularity, there were more than 170 gooseberry clubs in Britain and at least two formal clubs in the United States. The main purpose of a gooseberry club was to grow the largest, heaviest gooseberry. While most gooseberries are approximately the size and shape of an average green grape, some of the early prizewinners were the size of small plums.

MAIN DISH SALADS

ALPHA OMEGA SALAD

MAKES 2 SERVINGS

For a salad to work as a midday meal, it must contain protein and enough high-quality calories to feed both your body and your brain. This one does just that. With brain-boosting salmon, avocado, walnut, and chia (hello, omega-3s!), plus immunity-boosting spinach, blueberries, and onion, you'll feel nourished and energized.

- 4 cups (120 g) mixed greens, baby arugula, or baby spinach
- 1 cup (150 g) blueberries
- ¼ cup (30 g) chopped walnuts
- 2 tablespoons hemp seeds
- ½ red onion, thinly sliced
- 8 ounces (225 g) smoked salmon, chopped
- 1 Hass avocado, peeled and diced
- ⅓ cup (80 ml) avocado, walnut, or extra-virgin olive oil
- 3 tablespoons lemon juice
- 1 tablespoon chia seeds
- 1 tablespoon coconut nectar or honey
- Salt and pepper, to taste

1. In a large bowl, gently toss together the greens, berries, walnuts, hemp seeds, onion, salmon, and avocado. Set aside.

2. In a small bowl, whisk together the oil, lemon juice, chia seeds, coconut nectar, salt, and pepper.

3. Pour the mixture over the salad ingredients and toss, gently, once more.

SUPERFOOD SALAD

MAKES 2 SERVINGS

This is an outrageously superfood-filled salad that contains protein-packed quinoa, antioxidant-powered goji berries, fiber, omega-3-rich kale and sunflower seeds, garlic, and apple cider vinegar. You will feel so energized after eating this! Go ahead and make it ahead of time: It keeps beautifully for up to three days.

½ cup (55 g) dried goji berries soaked
   for twenty minutes or more in ½ cup of
   room-temperature water

3 cups (510 g) cooked red or white quinoa

1 large head curly leaf kale, washed,
   and ribs removed from leaves

1 cup (140 g) sunflower seeds

2 tablespoons apple cider vinegar

2 teaspoons whole-grain, brown, Dijon, or
   honey mustard

6 tablespoons extra-virgin olive oil

2 garlic cloves, minced

Salt and pepper, to taste

1. When you're ready to use the berries, drain the water (save it to drink; it's healthy!) and pat the berries dry with paper towels or a clean dish towel. Set aside.

2. Add the cooked quinoa to a large bowl. Set aside.

3. Stack the kale leaves on top of each other and slice into ½-inch (1.25 cm) ribbons. Add to the quinoa.

4. Add the hydrated goji berries and sunflower seeds to the bowl.

5. In a small mixing bowl, whisk together the vinegar, mustard, olive oil, garlic, salt, and pepper, and pour over the kale-quinoa-goji berry mixture. Stir to combine.

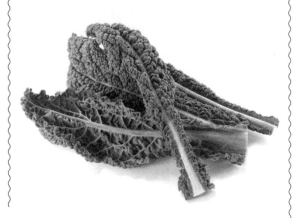

MULTI-BERRY LUNCHEON SALAD

MAKES 2 MAIN-DISH SERVINGS

You'll love this! Feel free to add chopped chicken, thin slices of pork, or fish if you want to increase the protein.

- ¼ cup (50 ml) raspberry vinegar
- ½ cup (125 ml) honey
- 1 clove garlic, minced
- Salt and pepper, to taste
- ⅛ teaspoon ground mustard seed
- ⅓ cup (80 ml) avocado, walnut, almond, or extra-virgin olive oil
- 8 ounces (225 g) baby spinach
- 8 ounces (225 g) butter lettuce
- 4 green onions (scallions), trimmed and sliced
- 1 cup (165 g) strawberries, sliced
- ½ cup (60 g) raspberries
- ½ cup (70 g) blackberries
- 1 cup (150 g) blueberries
- 1 cup (110 g) slivered almonds, toasted

1. In a small bowl, whisk together the vinegar, honey, garlic, salt, pepper, and mustard, until blended. Keep whisking and slowly pour in the oil, whisking until completely emulsified.

2. In a large bowl, toss together the remaining ingredients.

3. Drizzle the vinaigrette over the salad and toss once more, gently, to blend.

AUTUMN SALAD

MAKES 2 SERVINGS

The dried goji berries give this salad a chewy, slightly tart note that beautifully offsets the earthy flavor of winter squash.

- 1¾ cups (245 g) butternut squash, peeled and cubed
- 2 teaspoons plus 6 tablespoons walnut or extra-virgin olive oil, divided
- Salt and pepper, to taste
- 2 large handfuls baby spinach, arugula, or other salad leaves
- 1 tablespoon fresh parsley
- 2 cups (525 g) cannellini or other white beans, well drained
- ¼ cup (25 g) walnuts, chopped
- 2 tablespoons dried goji berries soaked for twenty minutes or more in ½ cup of room-temperature water
- 3 tablespoons balsamic vinegar
- 1 teaspoon Dijon or whole-grain mustard
- Salt and pepper, to taste

1. Preheat oven to 350°F (175°C or gas mark 4).

2. Place the butternut squash in a large bowl. Drizzle on 2 teaspoons walnut or extra-virgin olive oil and sprinkle with salt and pepper. Using your (clean) hands, toss the butternut squash until thoroughly coated with oil and season with salt and pepper, to taste. Place in a roasting pan and bake for up to thirty minutes, or until fork-tender, turning the squash once or twice during roasting.

3. Remove the butternut squash from the oven and let cool to room temperature.

4. In a large bowl, toss together the spinach or salad leaves, parsley, beans, walnuts, and cooled squash.

5. In a blender or food processor, process hydrated goji berries, remaining 6 tablespoons walnut or extra-virgin olive oil, vinegar, mustard, and salt, and pepper to taste, until smooth.

6. Adjust seasoning and toss with salad ingredients.

BERRY DRESSINGS

There are so many great, health-supportive dressings that contain berries that I could have created an entire cookbook devoted to them. Be warned, I may still do that one day, but for now I am limiting myself to some of my favorites, which you'll find here. All are filled with immunity-boosting berries and other nourishing ingredients.

MULBERRY SALAD DRESSING

MAKES ABOUT ½ CUP (125 ML)

1 cup (145 g) black mulberries

¼ cup (50 ml) orange juice

1 tablespoon balsamic vinegar

Salt and pepper, to taste

3 tablespoons extra-virgin olive oil

1. Add all the ingredients except the oil to a blender and process until smooth.

2. Gently pulse in the oil until the dressing is emulsified.

3. Refrigerate extra dressing in a covered container for up to five days.

GOJI STRAWBERRY VINAIGRETTE DRESSING

MAKES 1½ CUPS (350 ML)

This sprightly dressing is not only very high in vitamin C, but it's also great on everything from a green salad to mixed salad with chicken or shrimp.

- *½ cup (55 g) dried goji berries soaked for twenty minutes or more in 1½ cups of room-temperature water*
- *¼ cup (35 g) fresh or frozen strawberries*
- *¼ cup (50 ml) apple cider vinegar*
- *¼ cup (50 ml) balsamic vinegar*
- *1 teaspoon coconut nectar, honey, or sugar*
- *1 teaspoon ground mustard seed*
- *Salt and pepper, to taste*
- *¼ cup (50 ml) avocado oil or extra-virgin olive oil*

1. Drain the goji berries and drink the nutritious water or reserve it for another use.

2. Add all the ingredients except the oil to a blender and process until smooth.

3. Gently pulse in the oil until the dressing is emulsified.

4. Refrigerate extra dressing in a covered container for up to five days.

TANGY CRANBERRY SALAD DRESSING

MAKES 2½ CUPS (600 ML)

If you love pecans on your salad as much as I do, you must try this dressing. It pairs beautifully with pecans. It also works well with pork (try it drizzled over pork in a sandwich) and poultry.

- *1 cup (100 g) fresh cranberries*
- *1 medium navel orange, peeled and sectioned*
- *⅓ cup (80 ml) coconut nectar or honey*
- *½ cup (125 ml) apple cider vinegar*
- *1 teaspoon salt*
- *¼ teaspoon ground pepper*
- *1 teaspoon ground mustard seed*
- *1 teaspoon grated onion*
- *1 cup (250 ml) extra-virgin olive oil*

1. Add all the ingredients except the oil to a blender and process until smooth.

2. Gently pulse in the oil until the dressing is emulsified.

3. Refrigerate extra dressing in a covered container for up to five days.

GOLDEN BERRY SALAD DRESSING

MAKES ABOUT ⅔ CUP (160 ML)

If you love citrus-flavored dressings as much as I do, you'll love this antioxidant-rich version. Its bright, sunny taste pairs well with salads containing chicken, pork, or black beans.

1   cup (250 ml) orange juice

2   tablespoons dried golden berries

2   tablespoons avocado or extra-virgin olive oil

1   tablespoon almond or cashew butter

Salt and pepper, to taste

1. In a small saucepot, combine the orange juice and golden berries.

2. Over medium heat, bring the mixture to a boil, then reduce the heat and simmer the mixture uncovered for about ten minutes or until the mixture has reduced by about half. (The golden berries will look plump and float to top of mixture.)

3. Remove the mixture from the heat and allow it to cool.

4. Once cool, process the mixture with the oil, nut butter, salt, and pepper in a blender or food processor until smooth.

5. Refrigerate in an airtight container for up to five days.

BLUEBERRIES: DID YOU KNOW?

- Blueberry's white-gray waxy "bloom" is a protective coat.

- Early American colonists boiled blueberries with milk to make a gray-colored paint.

- Blueberries are the second most important commercial berry crop in the United States, with a total crop value of nearly $850.9 million in 2012.

- The United States is the world's largest producer of blueberries.

- Highbush Blueberries are the most commonly cultivated blueberries and the type found most often in grocery stores.

- Blueberries were not available, commercially until 1911, when Elizabeth White, the daughter of a New Jersey farmer, teamed up with USDA botanist Frederick Coville to identify wild plants with the most desirable properties, in order to crossbreed the bushes and create new, commercially viable blueberry varieties.

CREAMY ACAI DRESSING

MAKES 1⅔ CUPS (395 ML)

This creamy, protein-rich dressing tastes good on everything from a simple romaine lettuce salad to a shredded slaw. Acai berries have been said to do everything from squash colds and speed weight loss to cure cancer. While I can't guarantee all of those claims, it is safe to say that the tart taste of acai is delicious. You'll love this dressing.

1   cup (130 g) raw unsalted cashews

⅔   cup (160 ml) acai juice

2   tablespoons coconut vinegar or apple cider vinegar

2   teaspoons coconut nectar or honey

1   small garlic clove

Salt and pepper, to taste

1. Place the cashews in a small bowl and cover with water. Chill eight hours or overnight.

2. Drain the cashews and place them in a blender. Add the remaining ingredients and process until smooth, one to two minutes. If the dressing is too thick, add a tablespoon (or more) of acai juice or water.

3. Refrigerate extra dressing in a covered container for up to five days.

BOWLS

BLACK RICE BOWL

MAKES 2 SERVINGS

I don't eat a lot of rice—I find that it brings on wicked carb cravings—but I make an exception for black rice. Its satisfying chewy texture and high protein and fiber content leave me feeling satisfied, while its high antioxidant content makes me feel as if I am doing something great for my immune system. Add delicious berries, avocado, and nuts, and you have a deeply nourishing dish that is perfect for midday.

1½   cups (285 g) black rice

2¾   cups (620 ml) water

½   teaspoon salt

¼   cup (50 ml) freshly squeezed lime juice (from about 3 limes)

1½   tablespoons avocado or extra-virgin olive oil

1   clove garlic, minced

1   teaspoon coconut nectar or honey

2   tablespoons plus ½ cup, chopped fresh cilantro, divided

¼   teaspoon salt

Ground pepper, to taste

2   cups (290 g) fresh blackberries

1   *avocado, diced*

½   *cup (70 g) cashews or almonds, roughly chopped*

½   *cup (80 g) red onion, diced*

1. Rinse the rice in a mesh strainer and add to a medium saucepot with the water and salt. Bring to a boil over medium-high heat.

2. Cover the pot and reduce the heat to low. Allow the rice to simmer until done cooking, about thirty to forty minutes.

3. Remove the rice from the heat and cool.

4. Make the dressing by combining the lime juice, oil, garlic, coconut nectar, 2 tablespoons of cilantro, salt, and pepper in a food processor. Pulse until the ingredients are thoroughly combined.

5. Pour the dressing over the rice and toss gently to combine.

6. Fold in the blackberries, avocado, nuts, red onion, and the remaining cilantro, gently mixing to combine.

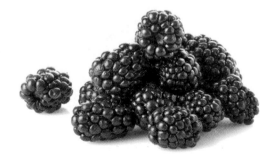

BLACK BEAN BLUEBERRY BOWL

MAKES 2 SERVINGS

This is an infinitely versatile recipe, one that you are welcome to customize as much or as little as you desire. If I have a jalapeno or red bell pepper in the house, I will add it to mix, and I've also added cubed pork tenderloin, pieces of shrimp or chicken, or increased the beans. It's all good!

1   *cup (150 g) blueberries*

Kernels from 2 cooked ears of corn

2   *cups (345 g) black beans, well drained*

2   *tablespoons chopped fresh cilantro or parsley (or a combination)*

2   *tablespoons extra-virgin olive oil*

1   *teaspoon balsamic vinegar*

½   *teaspoon salt*

Juice from ½ lime

1. In a large bowl, combine the blueberries, corn, black beans, and cilantro.

2. In a small bowl, whisk together the oil, vinegar, salt, and lime juice.

3. Pour the vinaigrette over ingredients in the large bowl and mix gently to combine.

QUINOA COCONUT CHICKEN BOWL

MAKES 2 SERVINGS

Quinoa, a "super seed" that we use as a culinary grain, is a high-protein wonder that not only leaves you feeling satiated, but also provides steady energy to help you get through whatever your workday throws at you too! Raspberries, red bell pepper, mango, and coconut make this salad especially delicious.

- 2   teaspoons plus 3 tablespoons liquid coconut oil, divided
- 2   cups (370 g) uncooked quinoa, rinsed
- 4   cups water
- 1   cup (370 g) diced mango
- 1   cup (125 g) raspberries
- ½   cup (80 g) red onion, diced
- 1   red pepper, diced
- ¼   cup (5 g) chopped fresh cilantro or parsley (or a combination)
- 1½ cups (125 g) unsweetened shredded coconut
- 1   cup (110 g) slivered almonds
- 2   cups (280 g) chopped cooked chicken, turkey, or pork or cooked black beans
- Juice of 5 limes
- Salt and pepper, to taste

1. Add 2 teaspoons of the coconut oil to a medium saucepot over medium-high heat. Add rinsed quinoa and stir until most of the moisture has evaporated.

2. Add 4 cups water to the quinoa. When it reaches a boil, cover the pot and turn the heat to low. Let it cook for fifteen to twenty minutes or until all water has been absorbed. Remove from the heat and allow the pot to sit, covered.

3. While the quinoa is cooking, combine the mango, raspberries, red onion, red pepper, cilantro, coconut, almonds, and chicken in a large bowl.

4. In a small bowl, whisk together the remaining 3 tablespoons of coconut oil, lime juice, salt, and pepper.

5. Add the quinoa and vinaigrette to the ingredients in the large bowl. Gently fold ingredients together, taking care not to crush the berries.

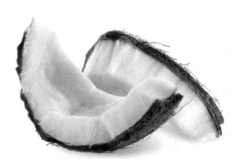

WRAPS & SANDWICHES

BERRY NUT BUTTER POCKET

MAKES 1 SERVING

This sandwich is a riff on the classic PB&J that many of us grew up with. Feel free to sneak in a few banana slices or some other not-too-juicy fruit, and switch in a different nut or seed butter if desired.

1 pita, split in half, preferably whole wheat, multigrain, or gluten-free

2 tablespoons almond butter or another nut or seed butter

1 tablespoon honey

¼ cup (35 g) blackberries, raspberries, or blueberries

1. Spread a layer of almond butter on the inside of each pita half.

2. Spread the honey directly over the almond butter.

3. Place the berries in a single layer over the almond butter and honey.

4. Optional: Warm the sandwich by grilling on a hot skillet or a panini press, about one minute on each side.

RED CURRANTS: DID YOU KNOW?

- A mature red currant bush can produce up to 9 pounds (4 kilograms) of fruit each summer.

- The large, sweet currants we know today were first grown commercially in Belgium and northern France in the seventeenth century.

- Red currants are known as *Johannisbeeren*, (John's berry) in Germany, because they begin to ripen around St. John's Day, also known as Midsummer Day, June 24.

- In German-speaking areas, red currant syrup or nectar flavors a soda called *Johannisbeerschorle*.

- This berry is popular flavor for iced drinks and desserts in Mexico.

- In movie making, red currant jelly is a popular stand-in for blood and blood-containing fluids.

- A compress of red currants is a traditional treatment for wounds that are not healing properly.

- Tea made from dried red currant leaves is a traditional treatment for rheumatism and gout.

AVOCADO-BEAN-BERRY SANDWICH

MAKES 1 SERVING

If something has avocado on it, I want to eat it. Which is why I love this sandwich. Yes, the strawberry-avocado combo sounds unusual, but you'll like it. Believe me. (If you'd like, add a few bits of last night's leftover chicken breast.)

¼ *avocado*

¼ *cup (65 g) cannellini or another white bean, well drained*

Salt and pepper, to taste

2 *slices sandwich bread, preferably whole grain or gluten-free, toasted*

¼ *cup (40 g) strawberries, sliced*

¼ *cup (10 g) baby spinach*

1. In a small bowl, mash together the avocado and cannellini beans, seasoning with the salt and pepper.

2. Spread the avocado-bean mixture on each slice of bread.

3. Layer the strawberries one slice of the bread. Top with the spinach leaves.

4. Put remaining the slice of bread on top and gently press together to "solidify" the sandwich.

BLUEBERRY CHICKEN SALAD SANDWICH

MAKES 4 SERVINGS

I first had fruit and chicken together in cherry-crazy Michigan, where I have relatives (hello, Ludington!). I loved the combination. Here, I pair poultry with dried cranberries, but feel free to experiment with other dried fruits.

⅓ *cup (60 g) cannellini beans, well drained*

¼ *cup (50 ml) avocado, walnut, pecan, or extra-virgin olive oil*

2 *tablespoons white wine vinegar*

Salt and pepper, to taste

4 *cups (560 g) cooked chicken, cubed*

1 *rib celery, finely diced*

2 *medium shallots, minced*

¾ *cup (90 g) blueberries*

½ *cup (55 g) pecans, coarsely chopped*

8 *slices sandwich bread, preferably whole grain or gluten-free*

1. Add the beans, oil, vinegar, salt, and pepper to a food processor. Process until creamy. Adjust the seasoning if necessary.

2. In a large bowl, combine the pureed beans with chicken, celery, shallots, dried cranberries, and pecans.

3. Cover and chill for twenty minutes to allow the flavors to combine.

4. Distribute the chicken salad among four bread slices. Top the salad with the remaining four bread slices and press down gently to "solidify" the sandwich.

PULLED PORK SURPRISE WRAP

MAKES 1 SERVING

When my family does eat meat, one of the things we enjoy is pulled pork. This sandwich came about when I was trying to do "something healthy" with leftovers.

1 12-inch (30-cm) sandwich wrap or tortilla, preferably whole grain or gluten-free, at room temperature

¼ cup (35 g) pulled pork or chicken (or barbecued brisket)

Optional: 1 or 2 tablespoons barbecue sauce

½ cup (70 g) blackberries

½ cup (35 g) baby kale leaves

1. Lay the wrap or tortilla on a flat surface.

2. Spread pork across the wrap, stopping an inch before the outer perimeter. Feel free to mix in a bit of barbecue sauce.

3. Sprinkle berries across the pork.

4. Lay the baby kale leaves over the berries.

5. To fold the wrap, think of it as the face of a clock. Fold in the sides located at the 3:00 and 9:00 positions, tucking them inward. Next, starting at the 6:00 position, begin rolling up toward the 12:00 position, making sure to tuck in the outer ends. Ingredients will fall out as you go—simply push everything back in and keep wrapping.

BERRY SANDWICH IDEAS

I rarely follow recipes for sandwiches. I go by what's in the kitchen, instead. But I do realize the power of suggestion, so I offer a few here:

- Hummus, chopped walnuts, dried goji berries, alfalfa sprouts, or baby greens
- White beans, chopped avocado, mulberries, and sunflower seeds
- Cashew butter, mulberries, and banana
- Hummus mixed with pumpkin puree, blackberries, and baby greens
- Roast beef, white bean spread, and red currants
- Sliced pork, cranberry sauce, and pecans
- Chopped cooked shrimp, moistened with coconut cream and lemon juice, blackberries, and cilantro

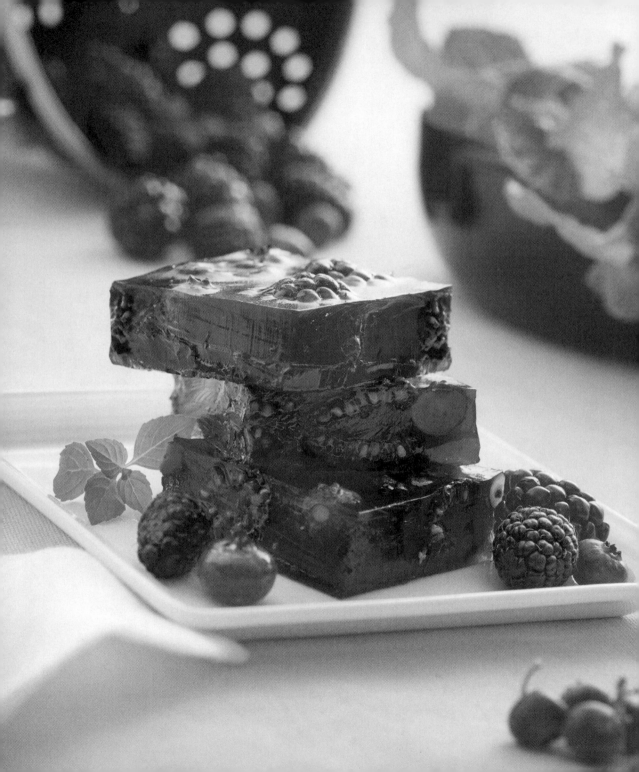

CHAPTER 6

BERRY SNACKS

I spent a good portion of my childhood in northern California, a place where blackberries grow wild. For my friends and me, berries were the ultimate snack food: We'd find a bramble of ripe berries, pick a few, and pop them into our mouths! I still love snacking on berries. But today I live in New York City, a place where there are no berry brambles to be found. So I head to my local fruit seller, farmers' market, or grocery store and purchase a few pints. If I'm lucky enough to have any extra fruit, I make one of these superfood-packed snacks. Each is an easy, delicious way to nourish the body using wholesome berries.

SWEET SNACKS

NO-BAKE BLUEBERRY-COCONUT BARS

MAKES 16 SERVINGS

Berry season is in the summer, a time when many of us refuse to turn on our ovens. This creamy, coconut-based blueberry bar allows you to stay cool while enjoying a superfood-packed treat.

- 2 cups (480 g) coconut butter (sometimes called coconut manna or creamed coconut)
- 2 cups (300 g) blueberries
- ¼ cup (50 ml) coconut nectar or Grade B maple syrup
- Optional: 1 teaspoon vanilla extract
- Optional: ½ teaspoon lemon zest

1. Line an 8-inch (20-cm) square baking pan with parchment paper or foil, leaving enough extra paper or foil on each side for easy removal of the finished bars. Set aside.

2. Combine all the ingredients in a food processor. Process until the mixture is smooth. It will be thick.

3. Spoon the mixture into the prepared pan, using a wet spatula to evenly spread the batter.

4. Refrigerate the pan for an hour or until the mixture is firm to the touch.

5. To cut, lift the bars out with the edges of the parchment paper, using a sharp knife to cut into squares.

6. Refrigerate or freeze leftovers for up to three months.

OPPOSITE: **Whole Berry Gelatin, page 114**

DIY CRANBERRY RAW FOOD BARS

MAKES 8 BARS

My kids love Lärabars™, those raw whole-food bars manufactured by Clif® Bar & Company. I love them too, but like many whole-food products, they are too pricey to enjoy regularly. Fortunately, this do-it-yourself version tastes just as delicious.

1½ cups (215 g) raw almonds or a mixture of almonds and cashews

1½ cups (180 g) dried unsweetened cranberries (not Craisins®)

Optional: 1 tablespoon hemp seeds

Optional: 1 tablespoon shredded coconut

8 to 10 Medjool dates (pits removed)

1. Line an 8-inch (20-cm) square baking pan with parchment paper or foil, leaving enough extra paper or foil on each side so the bars can be easily removed. Set pan aside.

2. In a food processor, combine nuts, dried cranberries, hemp seeds, coconut, and dates with ½ tablespoon of water. Pulse three or four times.

3. If the mixture is not yet clumping together, add another ½ tablespoon of water and pulse two or three times. Add a bit more water if needed and pulse a couple more times until the mixture clumps together.

4. Spoon the mixture into the prepared pan, using a wet spatula to press the mixture firmly into place.

5. Chill for an hour or until mixture is firm to the touch.

6. Once firm, use a pizza cutter to cut into bars.

7. Chill uneaten bars for up to five days.

WHY YOU SHOULD EAT DATES

Sweet, chewy, and satisfying, dates are one of the world's favorite fruits. Here are a few reasons for including them in your weekly diet:

- Dates contain high amounts of dietary fiber, which can help with everything from lowering cholesterol levels to improving digestion.

- The fruit contains flavonoid antioxidants that boast anti-inflammatory properties, while simultaneously strengthening the immune system and helping with healthy blood clotting.

- Dates contain Vitamin A, B-complex, and Vitamin K.

- They are rich in the minerals iron, potassium, calcium, manganese, copper, and magnesium.

NUT-FREE PROTEIN BITES

MAKES ABOUT 12 SERVINGS

These yummy nuggets are so easy to make—
and eat. I like to carry a few in my bag so
I have something to give hungry kids. Feel
free to try dried unsweetened cranberries or
another dried fruit in place of the dried goji
berries.

1½ cups (155 g) uncooked quinoa flakes
(These look like rolled oats and are
available in natural food stores.)

Dash of salt

2 tablespoons chia seeds

2 tablespoons hemp seeds

1 teaspoon ground ginger

½ teaspoon ground cinnamon

1 tablespoon dried goji berries

10 Medjool dates

2 tablespoons liquid coconut oil

1. Line a large baking sheet with wax paper.
Set aside.

2. In a food processor, combine the quinoa
flakes, salt, chia seeds, hemp seeds, ginger,
and cinnamon. Pulse three or four times.

3. Add in the goji berries, dates, and coconut
oil. Pulse three or four more times to
combine. The mixture should be starting to
clump together. If it is not, add ½ teaspoon

of water and pulse once or twice more. Add
more water as needed.

4. Wet your hands. Using a tablespoon of
mixture at a time, roll into a ball and place on
prepared baking sheet.

5. Chill the balls on baking sheet for an hour
or until they are firm.

6. Chill uneaten Protein Bites in a covered
container for up to five days.

BERRY BOMBS

MAKES 20 SERVINGS

This delicious snack features protein-rich
quinoa, sunflower seeds, cholesterol-lowering
oats, heart-healthy coconut, and super-
ingredient chia. Oh, and berries, too!

Optional: Liquid coconut oil to grease the pan

1 cup (80 g) old-fashioned oats

½ cup (85 g) cooked quinoa

½ cup (40 g) shredded unsweetened coconut

¼ cup (35 g) sunflower seeds

¼ cup (25 g) flax meal

2 tablespoons chia seeds

⅓ cup (80 ml) Grade B maple syrup

½ cup (60 g) dried unsweetened cranberries

¼ cup (25 g) dried blueberries

¼ cup (25 g) dried goji berries

(continued)

1. Preheat oven to 350°F (175°C or gas mark 4).

2. Grease the cups of a mini-muffin pan or line with mini-muffin papers. Set aside.

3. In a food processor, combine the oats, quinoa, coconut, sunflower seeds, flax meal, and chia seeds. Pulse two times to blend.

4. Add the maple syrup and pulse four or five times to blend.

5. Add the cranberries, blueberries, and dried goji berries and pulse two or three more times to blend.

6. Spoon the mixture evenly into each cup. Press down the mixture with your fingers.

7. Bake for eight to twelve minutes.

8. Let cool before removing from muffin tins. Store uneaten Berry Bombs in a covered container in the refridgerator for up to five days.

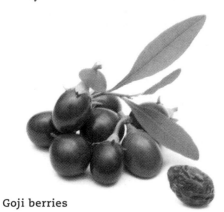

Goji berries

HOMEMADE VEGAN BLUEBERRY GRANOLA BARS

MAKES 8 BARS

Everyone needs a healthy granola bar recipe—something easy to make, filled with wholesome ingredients, and yummy. Consider this vegan version. Use dried unsweetened cranberries, dried goji berries, or another fruit if you'd like.

2   tablespoons chia seeds, ground (You can grind these in a spice or coffee grinder or a food processor,) and mixed with 4 tablespoons of water to form a gel

⅓   cup (80 ml) Grade B maple syrup

2½ cups (200 g) gluten-free old-fashioned oats

2   tablespoons hemp seeds

2   tablespoons sunflower seeds

1   teaspoon ground cinnamon or ginger, or a mix of the two

Dash of salt

⅓   cup (40 g) dried blueberries

1. Preheat oven to 350°F (175°C or gas mark 4).

2. Line a baking pan with parchment paper or foil, leaving enough extra paper or foil on each side so the bars can be easily removed.

3. In a large bowl, whisk together the chia gel and maple syrup. Set aside.

4. In another bowl, whisk together the remaining ingredients.

5. Add the dry ingredients to the wet ingredients and stir until thoroughly combined.

6. Spoon the mixture into the baking pan. With the back of a wet spatula, spread the mixture evenly.

7. Re-wet the spatula if needed and firmly press the mixture into place.

8. Bake for twenty minutes.

9. Let the pan completely cool before cutting into bars and removing from the baking pan.

THE MARVELS OF MAPLE

Maple syrup is the sweet sap of the sugar, black, and red maple trees, and it's a terrific sweetener to add to the health-supportive kitchen. That's because, ounce for ounce, maple contains fewer calories and more minerals than honey or sugar. Look for Grade B (sometimes called Dark Amber) maple syrup. It's darker and richer in taste than the lighter, less complex Grade A, or Light Amber, syrup. It also contains more of the manganese and zinc that maple is known for, two minerals essential for healthy immune system function.

FRUIT-ONLY LEATHER
MAKES 12 SERVINGS

I grew up eating a lot of homemade fruit leather. My mom made it, my grandmother made it, many of my friends' mothers made it. But the amount of sugar in most fruit leather recipes has always bothered me. I was thrilled to learn that you can make fruit leather without sugar! If this recipe is too tart for you, add a tablespoon or two of sugar or a few Medjool dates to the food processor. But try it without sweetener first. And yes, you can substitute other berries for the strawberries.

4 cups strawberries

1. Turn on the oven to its lowest temperature. (Ideal is 145°F (65°C), but many ovens don't go below 180°F (80°C) or 170°F (75°C).) If your oven has a convection option, go ahead and use it.

2. Line two baking sheets with parchment paper or silicone baking mats. Set aside.

3. Place the berries in a food processor or blender and process until they are a smooth paste.

4. Scrape the pureed berries onto the prepared baking sheets, using a wet spatula to spread

(continued)

the paste evenly, about ⅛- to ¼-inch (3-mm to 6-mm) thick, depending upon your preference. Leave a 1-inch border around the puree.

5. Bake for six to eight hours or until the fruit paste is shiny and slightly tacky to the touch. (If it is dry with no stickiness, the puree has overcooked, giving you fruit jerky instead of fruit leather. Fruit jerky still tastes good, but will take considerable work to eat.)

6. Allow the leather to cool to room temperature.

7. Slowly peel the cooled fruit leather away from the parchment paper. Using slightly oiled scissors to prevent sticking, cut the sheet into twelve or more strips, as narrow or thick as desired. Lay each strip on a piece of similarly sized wax paper and roll into a spiral. Store spirals in a covered container or plastic bag.

8. Store uneaten leather in a covered container or sealed bag at room temperature for up to a week.

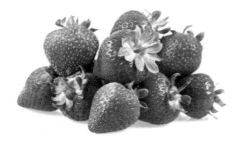

SUPER BERRY FRUIT LEATHER

MAKES 10 SERVINGS

This superfood berry fruit leather recipe features powdered white mulberry or goji berry, some chia, and applesauce or pear sauce. Yum!

3 tablespoons white mulberry powder or goji berry powder

2 cups (475 ml) unflavored applesauce or pear sauce (Feel free to replace one cup with your favorite pureed berries.)

2 tablespoons chia seeds

1. Turn oven on to its lowest temperature. (Ideal is 145°F (65°C), but many ovens don't go below 180°F (80°C) or 170°F (75°C).) Use convection if your oven has it.

2. Line a baking sheet with parchment paper or silicone baking mats. Set aside.

3. In a medium bowl, stir together white mulberry or goji powder and applesauce or pear sauce until completely combined.

4. Stir in chia seeds.

5. Scrape the mixture onto the prepared baking sheet, using a wet spatula to spread the mixture evenly, about ⅛- to ¼-inch (3-mm to 6-mm) thick, depending upon your preference. Leave a 1-inch border around the puree.

Do you remember the nursery rhyme "Here We Go Round the Mulberry Bush?" If you're one of the many people who have wondered why one would want to dance around a mulberry bush, it may have something to do with the ancient Celts, who believed that dancing around a mulberry tree at Summer Soltice would help protect them from malicious fairies.

6. Bake for six to eight hours or until the fruit paste is shiny and slightly tacky to the touch. (If it is dry with no stickiness, the paste has overcooked, giving you fruit jerky instead of fruit leather.) Fruit jerky still tastes good, but will take considerable work to eat.

7. Allow the leather to cool to room temperature.

8. Slowly peel the cooled fruit leather away from the parchment paper. Using slightly oiled scissors to prevent sticking, cut the sheet into ten or more strips, as narrow or thick as desired. Lay each strip on a piece of similarly sized wax paper and roll into a spiral.

9. Store uneaten leather in a covered container or sealed bag at room temperature for up to a week.

STRAWBERRY & ALMOND FRUIT ROLL-UPS

MAKES ABOUT 12 SERVINGS

This is a delicious protein-rich fruit roll-up. The almond butter gives it a PB&J taste. Your kids will love this! And yes, you absolutely can use a different nut butter or another berry in place of the strawberries.

2 cups (290 g) strawberries (You can also use blueberries, raspberries or blackberries, or a combination of these.)

½ cup (120 g) unflavored applesauce

2 Medjool dates, pitted

1 tablespoon almond butter

1. Turn oven on to its lowest temperature. (Ideal is 145°F (65°C), but many ovens don't go below 180°F (80°C) or 170°F (75°C).) If your oven has a convection option, go ahead and use it.

2. Line two baking sheets with parchment paper or silicone baking mats. Set aside.

3. Place all the ingredients in a food processor and process until they are a smooth paste.

4. Scrape the fruit paste onto the prepared baking sheets, using a wet spatula to spread the mixture evenly, about ⅛- to ¼-inch (3 mm to 6-mm) thick, depending upon your preference. Leave a 1-inch border around the paste.

(continued)

5. Bake for six to eight hours or until the fruit is shiny and slightly tacky to the touch. (If it is dry with no stickiness, the paste has overcooked, giving you fruit jerky instead of fruit leather.) Fruit jerky still tastes good, but will take considerable work to eat.

6. Allow the leather to cool to room temperature.

7. Slowly peel cooled fruit leather away from the parchment paper. Using slightly oiled scissors to prevent sticking, cut the sheet into ten or more strips, as narrow or thick as desired. Lay each strip on a piece of similarly sized wax paper and roll into a spiral.

8. Store uneaten leather in a covered container or sealed bag at room temperature for up to a week.

WHOLE BERRY GELATIN

MAKES 9 SERVINGS

This pretty gelatin is a favorite for two of my sons. They love the whole berries, which are suspended in the translucent base. Give it a try!

- 1 cup (125 g) whole berries (You can use one type or a mix.)
- ¼ cup (50 ml) cold water
- 2 tablespoons (2 pouches/envelopes) natural gelatin
- ¼ cup (50 ml) hot water (near boiling)
- 1⅓ cups (315 ml) unsweetened berry juice

1. Arrange the cut fruit or berries on the bottom of an 8-inch (20-cm) square heatproof glass pan, or something similar in size.

2. In a medium bowl, pour in the cold water. Sprinkle the powdered gelatin evenly over the water and soften for about eight minutes.

3. Whisk in the hot water until the gelatin is dissolved and fully incorporated.

4. Quickly whisk in the juice.

5. Gently, so as not to disrupt the berries, pour the mixture over the fruit. Cover the pan and chill for three hours or until the gelatin is fully set.

6. Cut into nine squares.

BLUE RASPBERRIES: DID YOU KNOW?

Ever wonder where blue raspberry flavor came from? A box of Otter Pops contained cherry, strawberry, watermelon, and raspberry treats, all requiring a different shade of red. Manufacturers decided to make cherry a dark red, strawberry a light red, watermelon a light pink, and raspberry a very dark red. But FD&C Red No. 2, the colorant used for raspberry-flavored food items, was banned in 1976, and food manufacturers needed a replacement. That's when some food scientists discovered blue raspberry. They took the flavor from the whitebark raspberry, which bears a blackish-bluish fruit, with a rarely used blue food dye called FD&C Blue No. 1. "Blue raspberry" was born. Today, it's a food-industry standard.

FROZEN SNACKS

FRUITY CHIA POPS

MAKES 6 SERVINGS

People often ask me how I get my kids to eat healthfully. Each parent has her own style: Mine is a combination of stealth, education, and coercion, used in different parts depending upon the individual kid. (Yes, each of my children has a different affinity—or tolerance—for healthy food.) This is one of my stealthier recipes, featuring antioxidant-generous berries, enzyme-rich pineapple, chia seeds that contain omega-3 fatty acids, and soluble fiber and protein as well as vitamins and minerals.

1   cup (250 g) frozen raspberries

1   cup (250 g) frozen pineapple or mango

⅓ cup (55 g) chia seeds

1   cup (250 ml) orange juice (You could also use your favorite berry juice, lemonade, or unsweetened coconut water.)

¼ cup (50 ml) water

1. Place all the ingredients in a food processor or blender. Process until completely smooth.

2. Pour the mixture into popsicle molds and freeze until solid, about three hours.

COCONUT BERRY POPS

MAKES 12 SERVINGS

This cool, creamy treat is a great option for people who are trying to wean themselves off of commercial ice cream and ice cream bars. Coconut milk gives these pops a luscious creaminess, and the berries add just the right touch of sweetness. Of course those ingredients also make and keep you healthy!

1 *13.5- to 15-ounce (415-ml) can, coconut milk*

6 *tablespoons coconut nectar, honey, or another natural sweetener*

¼ *cup (20 g) dried unsweetened coconut*

2 *cups (245 g) fresh or frozen berries (My favorite is a mix of raspberries, red currants, and strawberries.)*

Optional: A squirt or two of lemon juice or lime juice

1. Place all the ingredients in a food processor or blender. Process until completely smooth.

2. Fill the popsicle molds and freeze until solid, about three hours.

PERSONALIZE YOUR POPS

Feel free to customize the popsicle recipes in this book by substituting ingredients (different berries, for example, than the ones suggested) and adding one or more of the following:

• Toss ¼ to ½ cup (20 to 40 g) dried shredded coconut into the blender with your ingredients to create a denser, creamier ice pop.

• If your popsicles are melting too fast, add 1 to 2 teaspoons of unflavored gelatin powder to the liquid ingredients. This creates a slightly less icy popsicle, but it is great for slowing down what my kids call "the melties." (Plant-based gelatin powder is fine.)

• Shaved dark chocolate makes a fun addition for chocoholics.

• Want more protein? Toss in ½ cup (70 g) or more of your favorite nut or seed, either whole or chopped.

• If you don't like coconut milk, try cashew milk, hemp milk, or any other plant-based milk.

• If you want your pops to taste sweeter, puree half a ripe banana with the liquid ingredients.

• Like chewy textures? Fold in ½ cup (70 g) dried unsweetened cranberries or dried goji berries.

COCONUT WATER BERRY POPS

MAKES 6 SERVINGS

I just have to say it: This is a beautiful popsicle. It may not be super sweet, but it certainly is a cool, refreshing midday snack for kids and adults. I like to have one of these pops after an afternoon workout to replace lost fluid. I happen to like my popsicle crowded with fruit, but feel free to use more or less berries, depending on what you prefer.

Optional: 1 tablespoon of your favorite natural sweetener

Optional: A squirt or two of lemon juice or lime juice

3 *cups (700 ml) unsweetened coconut water*

1 *cup (150 g) whole blueberries (or another sweet berry)*

1 *cup (125 g) whole raspberries (or another sweet berry)*

1. If desired, whisk the sweetener and lemon juice into the coconut water. Set aside.

2. Place a selection of whole berries in the bottom of each popsicle mold.

3. Fill each popsicle mold with the coconut water and freeze until solid, about three hours.

FRUITY NUT BUTTER POPS

MAKES 8 SERVINGS

This is a high-protein popsicle featuring nut butter and chia—kind of like a PB&J sandwich in popsicle form. Coconut adds a gorgeous creaminess, while berries are the flavoring agent. These are a bit filling—perfect for a midday or midmorning snack.

2 *cups (305 g) chopped strawberries*

1 *tablespoon chia seeds*

2 *tablespoons coconut nectar or other natural sweetener*

1¼ *cups (300 ml) canned coconut milk, divided*

2 *tablespoons nut butter of your choice, at room temperature*

1. Place the strawberries, chia seeds, coconut nectar, and 1 cup (250 ml) of the coconut milk in a food processor or blender. Process until completely smooth.

2. In a medium bowl, whisk together the nut butter and ¼ cup (50 ml) of the coconut milk.

3. Divide the nut butter–coconut mixture evenly among popsicle molds. Using a small spatula or butter knife, spread the mixture inside the popsicle mold to cover the sides.

4. Gently pour the berry mixture into the popsicle molds. Freeze until solid, about three hours.

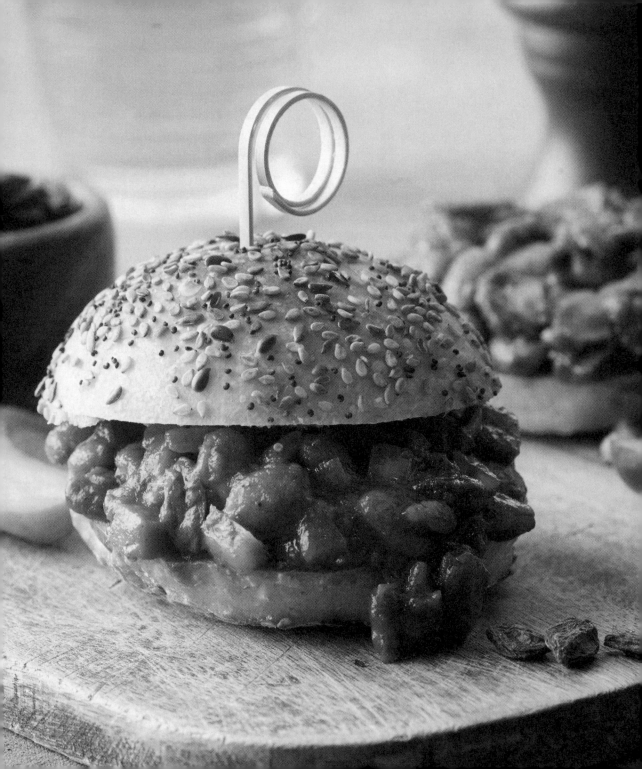

BERRIES FOR DINNER

For most of us, dinner is the big-deal meal of the day. We may skip breakfast and grab some random lunch food to wolf down or pick at while we are at our desk, but dinner is different. Not only is it the one meal most of us plan for, it's likely the one meal we never miss. Dinner is a time to leave our stressful work and school day behind and decompress. Anything that encourages people to slow down and enjoy their food is a very good thing, but you know how humans use food to self-soothe? Well, dinner is often when we do this by eating large volumes of starchy, fatty, comforting food. Not so good!

In this chapter, I am going to challenge you to rethink dinner as a time to do something wonderful for yourself. Incidentally, you'll notice that many of the recipes in this chapter are on the lighter side. There is a reason for this. I am not a fan of big dinners. Evening is typically a sedentary time, meaning your body doesn't need the large number of calories that a big meal contains; any calories that don't get burned are stored as fat. Also, undigested food impacts sleep. Here's to your health!

SALADS

BERRY MAIN-DISH SALAD BLUEPRINT

MAKES 2 SERVINGS

This is a recipe that can be played with in an infinite number of ways, so feel free to experiment and create something different at each meal!

- *6 cups (255 g) salad greens of your choice*
- *1 cup (125 g) berries of your choice*
- *2 cups (140 g) protein (chopped chicken, turkey, beef, pork, fish, shrimp, beans, lentils, etc.)*

(continued)

Optional: 1 cup (140 g) cooked grain (such as barley, millet, quinoa, or wild rice)

Optional: ¼ to ½ cup (30 g to 58 g) seeds or chopped nuts

Optional: ¼ to ½ cup (7 g to 15 g) chopped fresh herbs

Optional: ¼ cup (30 g) dried berries, such as unsweetened cranberries

1. Add all ingredients to a large bowl and gently toss to combine.

2. Dress with your favorite dressing and serve immediately. (Try the Berry Salad Dressing Blueprint.)

BERRY SIDE-DISH SALAD BLUEPRINT

MAKES 4 SERVINGS

Many of us grew up with "a salad on the side." Remember that ignored bowl of shredded iceberg that our moms put on the dinner table? Well, this is a blueprint for a "go with" salad that, I promise, will not be ignored!

4 cups (170 g) salad greens of your choice

1 cup (125 g) berries of your choice

Optional: ¼ cup (30 g) seeds or chopped nuts

Optional: ¼ cup (7 g) chopped fresh herbs

Optional: ¼ cup (30 g) dried berries, such as unsweetened cranberries

1. Add all ingredients to a large bowl and gently toss to combine.

2. Dress with your favorite dressing and serve immediately. (Try the following Berry Salad Dressing Blueprint.)

BERRY SALAD DRESSING BLUEPRINT

MAKES ½ CUP (125 ML)

This basic vinaigrette recipe can be customized in endless ways.

3 tablespoons raspberry vinegar or any other vinegar (such as apple cider, white wine, red wine, or balsamic)

¼ cup (30 g) berries of your choice or 2 tablespoons unsweetened cranberries or dried goji berries

1 teaspoon coconut nectar, coconut sugar, honey, or other sweetener

Salt and pepper, to taste

¼ cup (50 ml) hazelnut, almond, walnut, pecan, pistachio, or extra-virgin olive oil

1. Add everything but the oil to a blender and process until smooth.

2. Slowly add the oil, and process until the mixture is smooth and emulsified.

3. Store unused dressing in the refrigerator and use within three days.

SPICY STRAWBERRY GAZPACHO

MAKES 4 SERVINGS

If there are people you know who say they don't like gazpacho, this delicious, refreshing soup will convince them otherwise. Like other gazpachos, this one is bursting with antioxidants and fiber, making it a fantastic part of a heath-supportive diet.

- 2 cups (290 g) fresh or thawed frozen strawberries
- 1½ cups (365 g) fresh or high-quality canned tomatoes, diced
- 1 small cucumber, peeled and chopped
- 2 jalapeno chiles, seeded and chopped
- ¼ cup (10 g) mint leaves, chopped
- Juice of 2 limes
- 3 tablespoons coconut nectar or honey
- Salt and pepper, to taste

1. Place all the ingredients in a blender and puree until smooth.

2. Chill for twenty minutes before serving.

ALL THINGS RED GAZPACHO

MAKES 8 SERVINGS

Berries aren't typically the first ingredients that pop into your head when you think of soup, but they are brilliant in gazpacho! This version features your favorite red berries, plus beets and, yes, also tomatoes.

- 2½ cups (605 g) fresh or high-quality canned tomatoes, diced
- 2½ cups (305 g) red berries (a single type of berry or a mix of red currant, strawberry, raspberry, lingonberry, etc.)
- ½ cup chopped cooked red beet
- 1 garlic clove
- 1 small cucumber, peeled and chopped
- ½ cup (50 g) scallion, chopped (Go ahead and include as much green as you'd like.)
- ⅓ cup (50 g) green bell pepper, chopped
- ⅓ cup (80 ml) extra-virgin olive oil
- ⅓ cup (80 ml) sherry vinegar
- 1 teaspoon salt
- ½ teaspoon ground pepper

1. Add all the ingredients to a food processor or blender and pulse until blended to the consistency you enjoy. Pulse a few times for a chunky gazpacho. Or process until completely smooth. Adjust seasonings.

2. Chill for twenty minutes before serving.

GOJI BERRY SOUP

MAKES 4 SERVINGS

This flavorful soup is filled with powerful antibacterial, antiviral, and antifungal ingredients to help attack invading bacteria and viruses. And these ingredients are powerful immunity boosters that help your immune system fight off illness.

- 1 tablespoon liquid coconut or sesame oil
- 2 cups (140 g) sliced mushrooms
- 1 tablespoon minced fresh ginger
- 4 garlic cloves, minced
- 1 tablespoon red pepper flakes
- 4 cups (1 L) homemade chicken or vegetable broth
- 2 cups (280 g) shredded leftover cooked chicken (or cooked mung beans or lentils)
- 1 tablespoon soy sauce or fish sauce
- 1 tablespoon lemon juice
- 1 scallion, sliced (Feel free to use the green part too.)
- ¼ cup (30 g) dried goji berries, hydrated in a cup of warm water for twenty minutes

Salt and pepper, to taste

- 1 tablespoon chopped fresh cilantro or Thai basil (or a combination of the two)

1. Heat the oil in a saucepot over medium heat. Add the mushrooms and cook for two minutes or until they begin to soften.

2. Add the minced ginger, garlic, pepper flakes, and shredded chicken (or mung beans or lentils). Sauté for another minute or two until the ginger and garlic soften.

3. Add the broth, soy sauce, lemon juice, scallion, goji berries (go ahead and add their soaking water too), salt, and pepper. Allow to come to a boil.

4. Immediately turn off heat. Stir in the cilantro or Thai basil and adjust the seasonings.

BLACKBERRY SCRUB FOR FACE & BODY

MAKES ABOUT ½ CUP

This lovely scrub makes my skin look super glowy. The berries provide antioxidants, the honey is antibacterial, and the sugar provides scrubbing action.

- ⅓ cup blackberries
- 4 tablespoons raw honey
- 1 tablespoon raw or regular sugar

1. In a large bowl, mash the berries with the back of a fork or a potato masher.

2. Stir in the honey until smooth.

3. Add the sugar and mix well.

4. Use immediately. Scrub into clean skin in circular motion. For extra brightening, allow the mixture to sit on the skin for five to ten minutes before rinsing off with water.

VEGETARIAN MAIN DISHES

SMOTHERED SWEET POTATOES

MAKES 2 SERVINGS

This is my clients' favorite recipe. In each of my groups there's always someone who says, "So-and-so tells me I need to ask for your Smothered Sweet Potato recipe." It has several variations. This recipe features dried goji berries, an anti-inflammatory ingredient that supports a strong immune system and helps ward off illness. *Note:* You'll need to bake the sweet potatoes first, which can take up to an hour.

- 2 *medium sweet potatoes*
- 2 *cups (345 g) cooked black beans, rinsed*
- 1 *medium tomato, diced*
- ½ *tablespoon liquid coconut or extra-virgin olive oil*
- ½ *teaspoon ground cumin*
- ½ *teaspoon ground coriander*
- 2 *tablespoons fresh cilantro, chopped*
- *Salt and pepper, to taste*
- ½ *Hass avocado, diced*
- 2 *tablespoons hydrated goji berries*
- 2 *tablespoons sunflower seeds or pumpkin seeds*

1. Preheat oven to 425°F (218°C or gas mark 7).

2. Pierce the sweet potatoes with a fork in several places, place in a baking pan, and bake until tender all the way to the center, about one hour. Or cook in a microwave on high for eight to ten minutes, or until moderately soft.

3. While the sweet potatoes cook, add the beans, tomato, oil, cumin, coriander, cilantro, salt, and pepper to a medium saucepot over medium heat. Cook for three minutes.

4. Remove from the heat and allow the bean mixture to cool slightly.

5. When the sweet potatoes are done and have cooled just enough so you can handle them, cut the top of each lengthwise. Pry each sweet potato open and create a hollow that is large enough to contain the bean mixture.

6. Divide the black bean mixture between the two potatoes. Top with the avocado, goji berries, and seeds.

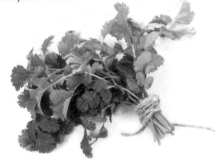

SLOW COOKER BERRY-BEAN SLOPPY JOES

MAKES ABOUT 10 SERVINGS

I am always looking for healthy slow-cooker recipes that my family will like. I think this is a winner! If you don't have ten people to feed, go ahead and freeze the extras.

2   tablespoons extra-virgin olive oil, plus extra for coating the slow cooker

1   large white onion, diced

2   medium carrots, diced

1   large red, yellow, or orange bell pepper, diced

1   jalapeno or serrano chile, deseeded and minced

5   cloves garlic, minced

2   tablespoons chili powder

2   tablespoons apple cider vinegar

2   cups (385 g) dry pinto beans, soaked overnight

½   cup (55 g) dried goji berries

1   8-ounce (225 g) can tomato sauce

½   cup (125 ml) vegetable broth or water

2   tablespoons reduced-sodium soy sauce or tamari

1   6-ounce (170 g) can tomato paste

3   tablespoons prepared mustard, any style, such as Dijon, coarse, brown, or yellow

1   tablespoon honey

1   teaspoon salt

Ground pepper, to taste

10   whole-wheat hamburger buns

1. Heat 2 tablespoons of the oil in a large skillet over medium-high heat. Add the onion, carrots, and bell pepper and cook, stirring occasionally, until the vegetables start to brown, about eight minutes.

2. Stir in the chile, garlic, and chili powder and cook for about one minute.

3. Remove from the heat, stir in vinegar, and scrape up any browned bits.

4. Coat a 6-quart (6.5 L) slow cooker with olive oil.

5. Drain and rinse the soaked beans and transfer them and the goji berries to the slow cooker.

6. Stir in the tomato sauce, broth, tomato paste, soy sauce, mustard, honey, salt, and pepper to combine.

7. Spread the carrot-onion mixture directly on top of the bean mixture, being careful not to stir it into the beans.

8. Cover and cook on high for five hours or low for nine hours.

9. Serve the mixture on buns with your favorite condiments.

EDAMAME STRAWBERRY STEW

MAKES ABOUT 6 SERVINGS

This fresh-tasting stew is almost like a succotash. It provides protein, fiber, minerals, vitamins, phytonutrients, and healthy fats—everything your body needs to be its healthiest!

1½ 10-ounce (425 g) packages frozen shelled edamame (about 3 cups), thawed

1 tablespoon extra-virgin olive oil

1 large onion, chopped

1 large zucchini or crookneck squash, diced

1 large red bell pepper, diced

1 cup fresh or frozen corn kernels

2 tablespoons minced garlic

2 teaspoons ground cumin

1 teaspoon ground coriander

Salt and pepper, to taste

1 28-ounce (795 g) can diced tomatoes (with juice)

¼ cup (5 g) chopped fresh cilantro, parsley, or mint (or a combination)

1 cup (145 g) chopped strawberries

3 tablespoons lemon juice

1. Bring a large saucepot of water to a boil. Add the edamame and cook until tender, four to five minutes. Drain in a colander. Set aside.

2. Heat the oil in a large saucepot over medium heat. Add the onion and cook about three minutes or until starting to soften, stirring occasionally.

3. Add the squash, red bell pepper, and corn and cook, covered, until the vegetables soften and the onions begin to get golden, about three minutes.

4. Add the garlic, cumin, coriander, salt, and pepper and cook, stirring, until fragrant, about thirty seconds.

5. Raise the heat to medium-high and stir in the tomatoes. Bring to a boil and then reduce the heat to medium and simmer the stew for about five minutes, or until slightly reduced.

6. Stir in the edamame and cook until heated through, about two minutes more.

7. Remove from the heat and stir in the cilantro, strawberries, and lemon juice.

8. Allow the stew to sit for ten minutes before serving to allow the flavors to develop.

ACORN SQUASH WITH WALNUTS & CRANBERRIES

MAKES 2 SERVINGS

Stuffed acorn squash is a vegetarian favorite. It's yummy, it's healthy, and it's fun. This high-protein version features walnuts and white beans with cranberries. If you have leftover millet or quinoa on hand, use 2 cups (360 g) of that instead of the beans.

- 2 tablespoons Grade B maple syrup
- 2 tablespoons extra-virgin olive oil, divided
- ¼ teaspoon dried sage
- Salt and pepper, to taste
- 2 cups (360 g) white beans
- ½ cup (50 g) walnuts or pecans, roughly chopped
- ½ cup (50 g) fresh cranberries
- 1 acorn squash, cut in half, seeds removed

1. Preheat oven to 375°F (190°C or gas mark 5).

2. In a small bowl, whisk together the maple syrup, one tablespoon of the oil, sage, salt, and pepper.

3. In a large bowl, combine the beans, walnuts, and cranberries and the maple syrup mixture.

4. Rub the squash halves with the remaining olive oil. Sprinkle cut surfaces with salt and pepper and fill cavities with the bean-nut-berry mixture.

5. Place the squash halves in a baking pan, cover with foil, and bake for about an hour, or until the squash is soft.

BLACK CURRANTS: DID YOU KNOW?

- Cultivation of black currants, as a crop, is comparatively recent, occurring within the last 400 to 500 years.

- Black currant seed oil is used to treat a variety of skin conditions, such as eczema.

- Some people apply black currant leaf directly to the skin for treating wounds and insect bites.

- Black currants contain three times more vitamin C than an orange, helping them prevent joint inflammation, eyestrain, and urinary infections.

- Blackcurrants once grew abundantly in the United States, but in the early 1900s, the federal government banned cultivation of the berry because they were thought to facilitate white pine blister rust—a threat to the US lumber industry.

MEATY MAIN DISHES

BLUEBERRY SLIDERS

MAKES 4 SERVINGS

This is a fruity take on the ever-popular slider. Feel free to try another berry in place of the blueberries or use a mix of berries.

2   slices bread, preferably whole grain
    or gluten-free
¼   cup (50 g) walnuts
½   cup (75 g) fresh or frozen and thawed
    blueberries
1   tablespoon balsamic vinegar
2   teaspoons Dijon mustard
2   cloves garlic, minced
Salt and pepper, to taste
12 ounces (340 g) 90 percent lean ground beef
4   slider rolls

1. Place the bread and walnuts in a food processor and pulse into fine crumbs. Transfer to a large bowl.

2. Add the berries, vinegar, mustard, garlic, salt, and pepper to the food processor and pulse until pureed. Add the blueberry mixture to the bread-walnut crumbs.

BERRY COCONUT AGE-FIGHTING MASK

MAKES ABOUT ¼ CUP

Berries are high in antioxidants, which help prevent premature aging. This mask contains berries plus nourishing coconut oil and healing honey. Try this if you have normal to dry skin.

2 tablespoons liquid coconut oil
2 tablespoons raw organic honey
¼ cup mixed berries

1. Combine all the ingredients in a food processor and pulse until smooth.

2. Use immediately. Apply to clean skin and let sit on the skin for 20 minutes before before rinsing off with warm or cool water.

3. Add the beef to the bread-blueberry mixture and incorporate ingredients with your hands or a potato masher.

4. Form the mixture into eight patties, about 2 inches (5 cm) in diameter and a ½-inch (1.25-cm) thick.

5. To cook, brush a skillet, indoor or outdoor grill, or broiler pan with oil. Cook the patties via your desired method until they are cooked through, about four minutes per side.

6. Serve on slider rolls with your favorite condiments.

BERRY PORK CHOPS

MAKES 4 SERVINGS

This lovely combo features pork chops with blueberry sauce, though you're free to use blackberries or mulberries if you'd like.

3   tablespoons extra-virgin olive oil, divided

1   small red onion, thinly sliced

3   cups (445 g) fresh or frozen blueberries

2   tablespoons honey or Grade B maple syrup

Juice of 1 lemon

1   teaspoon fresh thyme leaves

Salt and pepper, to taste

4   bone-in, ½-inch (1.25-cm) thick pork chops (7 ounces, 200 g each)

1. In a large skillet, heat 1 tablespoon olive oil over medium-low heat. Add the onion and cook until softened, about five minutes.

2. Stir in the blueberries, honey, lemon juice, thyme, salt, and pepper. Simmer for five minutes, or until the blueberries have released their juices and the sauce has thickened.

3. Brush the pork chops with 2 tablespoons olive oil and season with salt and pepper. Grill the chops on a barbecue or pan-fry them over medium-high heat, about seven or eight minutes on each side.

4. Serve pork chops topped with blueberry sauce.

TURKEY TENDERLOIN WITH CRANBERRY-SHALLOT SAUCE

MAKES 6 SERVINGS

This holiday favorite is actually just as delicious as a non-holiday meal. It's healthy, too, thanks to infection-fighting shallots and cranberries (in two forms) and dried goji berries.

2   turkey tenderloins (about 1½ pounds [680 g] total)

Salt and pepper, to taste

1½ tablespoons extra-virgin olive oil, divided

4   shallots, minced

2   teaspoons chopped thyme

¾   cup (175 ml) chicken broth

1½ cups (150 g) fresh or frozen (not thawed) cranberries

¼   cup (30 g) dried cranberries or blueberries

¼   cup (28 g) dried goji berries

2   tablespoons Grade B maple syrup or honey

1   tablespoon raspberry vinegar

1. Preheat oven to 450°F (230°C or gas mark 8).

2. Sprinkle the turkey tenderloins with salt and pepper. Heat 2 teaspoons olive oil in a large skillet over medium heat. Add the turkey and cook, using tongs to turn the turkey to brown all sides. This should take about five minutes.

3. Transfer the turkey to a baking sheet and bake uncovered until an instant-read thermometer registers 165°F (74°C), about eighteen to twenty-four minutes.

4. Meanwhile, add the remaining olive oil to the pan. Add the shallots and cook, stirring occasionally, until browned, three minutes.

5. Add the thyme and cook just until fragrant, about ten seconds.

6. Add the broth and cook for one minute, scraping up any browned bits as you stir.

7. Stir in the fresh and dried cranberries and goji berries and cook for about six minutes, or until most of the fresh cranberries have broken down. Stir in the maple syrup, vinegar, and a bit of salt and pepper into the sauce and cook for one minute. Cover and remove from the heat.

8. For easier slicing, allow the just-cooked turkey to cool for five minutes before slicing.

9. To serve, slice the turkey thinly and drape with the sauce.

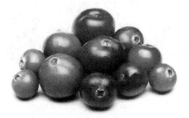

CHICKEN WITH BERRY SAUCE
MAKES 4 SERVINGS

The light, neutral taste of chicken breast pairs beautifully with most berries. Here, it teams up with antioxidant-rich blackberries. If you've got raspberries on hand, use them instead.

½ teaspoon ground cumin

¼ teaspoon ground allspice

¼ teaspoon salt

¼ teaspoon ground pepper

1¼ pounds (565 g) chicken cutlets

1   tablespoon extra-virgin olive oil

3   cups (430 g) blackberries

¼ cup (50 ml) chicken broth or water

1. In a small bowl, whisk together the cumin, allspice, salt, and pepper.

2. Rub 1 teaspoon of the spice mixture into chicken cutlets.

3. Heat the oil in a large skillet over medium heat. Add the chicken to the pan and cook about eight minutes, turning over once. (Do not wash the skillet.)

4. Transfer the chicken to a plate.

5. Add blackberries to the skillet—still over medium heat—and gently crush them to

(continued)

release their juice. Scrape up brown bits from the chicken. Add the broth and the rest of the spice mixture and cook for three minutes or until slightly reduced.

6. To serve, spoon the blackberry sauce over the chicken cutlets.

CURRIED HALIBUT WITH RASPBERRY-MANGO RELISH

MAKES 4 SERVINGS

This easy recipe is a fun way to eat fish. Plus, it's easy and kids love it. You'll need an oven-safe skillet for this recipe.

1 cup (125 g) chopped raspberries

1 cup (165 g) chopped mango

¼ cup (5 g) chopped fresh cilantro leaves, plus more for garnish

¼ cup (40 g) chopped red onion

¼ cup (20 g) unsweetened shredded coconut

2 teaspoons lime juice

4 to 5 teaspoons liquid coconut oil, divided

Salt and pepper, to taste

1½ pounds (680 g) halibut, skin trimmed, cut into 4 pieces, room temperature

1 tablespoon mild curry powder

1 13½-ounce (405 ml) can reduced-fat coconut milk

1. Place an oven-safe skillet in the oven and turn the oven to 500°F (260°C or gas mark 10).

2. In a large bowl, toss the raspberries, mango, cilantro, onion, coconut, lime juice, and 2 teaspoons of the coconut oil together. Season with salt and set the relish aside.

3. Generously season the fish with the curry powder and salt.

4. Heat the rest of the coconut oil in a large sauté pan over medium-high heat. Sear fish on both sides until golden brown, about forty-five seconds per side.

5. Transfer the fish to the hot skillet in the oven and roast until the fish is barely cooked through, about six more minutes. The flesh will feel firm and an instant-read thermometer inserted in the center of each piece should read 135°F (57°C). The fish will continue to cook when it comes out of the oven. Transfer it to a serving platter and top with raspberry-mango relish.

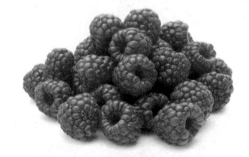

MAKE YOUR OWN
APPLE OR PEAR SAUCE

Need applesauce or pear sauce in a pinch? Both are quick to make at home. Here's how:

1. Take one large apples or two pears (you can use more if you'd like). One large apple or two pears will yield about 1 cup of applesauce. Peel apple or pears. Slice or chop fruit into any size pieces you'd like.

2. Place fruit into a small saucepot and add 2 or 3 tablespoons of water. Optional: Add a squirt of lemon juice, a sprinkle of ground cinnamon, or a drizzle of honey. Cook on medium-low heat until the apple or pear breaks down. (Add more water if the pot looks dry; you don't want the fruit to scorch.)

3. Puree cooked fruit and any liquid in the pot, using a food processor or blender, until smooth.

4. Store unused sauce in a covered container in the refrigerator for up to a week.

FRUITY SALMON

MAKES 2 SERVINGS

Many of my clients love salmon. Rich in omega-3 fatty acids, salmon is a great choice for anyone looking to improve brain and heart health. This fun version features three of the world's most popular berries: raspberry, blueberry, and strawberry. This is one of the easiest recipes in the book!

2 *tablespoons liquid coconut oil*

¼ *cup (40 g) diced sweet onion,
    such as Walla Walla or Vidalia*

8 *ounces (225 g) salmon steaks or fillets*

1 *cup (15 g) sugar peas or snow peas*

¼ *cup (30 g) raspberries*

¼ *cup (35 g) blueberries*

¼ *cup (40 g) sliced strawberries*

2 *tablespoons orange juice*

1. Heat the coconut oil in a large sauté pan over medium heat. Add the onions and cook until soft and just golden, about five minutes

2. Add the salmon and snow peas, cooking for about one minute on each side.

3. Add the berries and orange juice and cook for another five or six minutes, or until salmon is cooked through.

BERRY DINNER SAUCES

With their bright, complex flavors, berry-based dinner sauces are an easy and upscale way to add a healthy dose of nutrients to your dinners. Here are a few of my favorites.

ELDERBERRY SAUCE
MAKES 1½ CUPS (350 ML)

Elderberries are well known in the healing community for their ability to ward off colds. Here, they are made into a tangy sauce that's fantastic on poultry, meats, and grains.

*1½ cups (220 g) elderberries,
    completely de-stemmed*
¼ medium onion (30 g), chopped
¼ cup (50 ml) white wine vinegar
¼ cup (50 ml) honey
⅛ teaspoon ground allspice
⅛ teaspoon ground cloves
1/16 teaspoon ground cinnamon
1/16 teaspoon cayenne pepper
Salt and pepper, to taste

1. Add the elderberries, onion, and vinegar to a medium saucepot over medium-high heat. Bring to a boil, then reduce heat to medium and simmer for ten minutes.

2. Allow the mixture to cool slightly and add to a food processor or blender. Process until smooth.

3. Return the mixture to the saucepot, set the heat to medium-high, and add the remaining ingredients. Allow the mixture to boil.

Immediately reduce the heat to medium-low and allow the sauce to simmer for ten minutes, stirring frequently.

4. Allow the sauce to cool for ten minutes before using.

5. Refrigerate unused sauce in a covered container for up to two weeks.

BLACK CURRANT SAUCE
MAKES 2 CUPS (475 ML)

This beautiful sauce features the charms of fresh black currants. It works beautifully with fatty poultry (such as duck and goose) and game, but also works with pork, beef, salmon, and chicken. (I even like this black currant sauce over roasted mushrooms.) Like other berries, currants contain high amounts of vitamin C (three times more than oranges) and other anti-inflammatory ingredients. They also contain phenolic compounds, which help prevent and treat urinary tract conditions.

1 cup (250 ml) chicken stock
1 shallot, peeled and minced
1 teaspoon thyme leaves, minced
3 cups (335 g) black currants
1 tablespoon honey

*½ cup (125 ml) balsamic or apple cider
vinegar*

Salt and pepper, to taste

1. Add the chicken stock to a medium
saucepot over medium-high heat. Simmer
continually until the chicken stock has reduced
by about half. You can eyeball this—it doesn't
have to be exact.

2. Add the shallot and cook until the shallot
is soft. Continue to reduce the broth for three
more minutes.

3. Add the thyme leaves, black currants, honey,
and vinegar and simmer the sauce over low
heat for seven to ten minutes or until the black
currants have softened.

4. Using the back of a fork, smash the currants
against the side of the pot. You can use the
back of a wooden spoon to press against the
berries to crush them lightly.

5. Adjust the salt and pepper and allow the
sauce to cool for ten minutes before using.

6. You can leave the sauce chunky, or puree it
in a blender or food processor.

7. Refrigerate unused sauce in a covered
container for up to five days.

LINGONBERRY SAUCE
MAKES 3 CUPS (700 ML)

Lingonberries have been enjoyed for centuries
as both a food and a remedy. In folk medicine,
they've been used as a treatment for urinary
tract infections; a disinfectant; and a treatment
for diabetes, obesity, gout, arthritis, and viral
infections. Here, they bring their sweet-tart
charm to a lovely sauce that is great with pork,
beef, meatballs, chicken, turkey, goose, salmon,
grains, and so much more.

1 cup (250 ml) chicken or vegetable broth
½ cup (125 ml) honey
4 cups (400 g) lingonberries
Salt and pepper, to taste

1. Add the broth and honey to a medium
saucepot set over medium-high heat. Bring to
a boil and add the berries.

2. Immediately reduce heat to medium and
simmer for ten minutes.

3. Using the back of a fork or a potato masher,
gently mash some of the berries to thicken the
sauce.

4. Remove sauce from heat, stir in the salt
and pepper, and allow the sauce to cool for ten
minutes.

5. Refrigerate unused sauce in a covered
container for up to two weeks.

RED CURRANT SAUCE

MAKES 1½ CUPS (350 ML)

Fresh red currants are beautiful, tart, and very high in vitamin C and anti-inflammatory compounds, which help preserve eyesight, protect the heart and nervous system, help improve the complexion and support the immune system. This sophisticated sauce goes well with poultry, beef, and pork and also tastes great drizzled over grains.

1   pint (225 g) red currants (or 3 cups frozen red currants)
½   cup (125 ml) water or chicken broth
⅓   cup (80 ml) honey
2   tablespoons sherry vinegar
Salt and pepper, to taste

1. Add all the ingredients to a large saucepot over medium-high heat. Bring to a boil, then quickly lower the heat to medium and simmer the mixture, stirring frequently for ten minutes or until currants are soft.

2. Using the back of a large fork or a potato masher, mash the currants until they are broken and the sauce is thick. Remove from the heat.

3. You can leave the sauce chunky, or puree it in a blender or food processor.

4. Allow the sauce to cool for about ten minutes before using.

5. Refrigerate unused sauce in a covered container for up to five days.

GOOSEBERRY SAUCE

MAKES ABOUT 2 CUPS (475 ML)

Gooseberry sauce is refreshingly tart and rich in vitamin C. In the UK, it's traditionally enjoyed with game, poultry, and other meats, but I like to drizzle it over grains and potatoes as well as roasted veggies.

1   cup (250 ml) beef or chicken broth
1   tablespoon extra-virgin olive oil
2   tablespoons honey
1   pint (300 g) green gooseberries, rinsed and stems removed
Salt and pepper, to taste

1. Combine the broth, oil, and honey in a medium saucepot over medium-high heat. Allow the ingredients to simmer, stirring to dissolve the honey.

2. Add the gooseberries and simmer for about five more minutes or until gooseberries become soft. Using the back of a large fork or a potato masher, mash berries against the side of the pot, until a thick, creamy puree has appeared.

3. Remove from the heat and add salt and pepper. Allow to cool slightly before using.

4. Refrigerate unused sauce in a covered container for up to five days.

GRAIN SIDES

BERRY RED QUINOA PILAF

MAKES 6 SERVINGS

Red quinoa is the antioxidant-rich cousin of white quinoa. Use regular quinoa here if you'd like.

- *1½ cups (350 ml) chicken or vegetable broth*
- *¾ cup (130 g) red quinoa*
- *⅛ teaspoon ground pepper*
- *½ cup (30 g) finely chopped fresh parsley*
- *½ cup (60 g) chopped walnuts*
- *½ cup (60 g) dried unsweetened cranberries or dried blueberries*
- *1⅓ cups (165 g) raspberries, blackberries, mulberries, or black currants*

1. In a medium saucepot over medium-high heat, combine the broth, quinoa, and pepper. Bring to a boil.

2. Reduce heat to low, cover, and simmer twelve to fifteen minutes or until liquid is absorbed.

3. Let mixture cool for ten minutes before fluffing with a fork.

4. Transfer quinoa to a serving dish and gently fold in the parsley, walnuts, cranberries, and raspberries.

BERRY KALE QUINOA

MAKES 8 SERVINGS

I am always looking for great dishes— that are nutritious and just intriguing enough to pique people's interest—to take to potlucks, picnics, and cookouts. This is one of those dishes. It features protein-heavy quinoa, omega-3–heavy kale, and antioxidant-rich blueberries (though you're welcome to substitute another berry).

- *3 cups (555 g) cooked quinoa, cooled*
- *1 cup (150 g) blueberries*
- *1½ cups (100 g) shredded kale*
- *1 cup (90 g) sliced almonds or chopped walnuts*
- *3 tablespoons extra-virgin olive oil*
- *4 tablespoons lemon juice*
- *1 teaspoon honey or Grade B maple syrup*
- *1 small shallot, minced*
- *Salt and pepper, to taste*

1. In a large bowl, combine the quinoa, blueberries, kale, and almonds. Mix until well combined.

2. In a small bowl, whisk together the oil, lemon juice, honey, shallot, salt, and pepper. Pour it over quinoa mixture. Adjust the seasoning and allow mixture to sit for twenty minutes to blend flavors before serving.

HERBAL BERRY MILLET

MAKES 6 SERVINGS

Millet is a fantastic super seed that is rich in protein, vitamin B₆, iron, and magnesium. Unfortunately, it is a bit bland and requires a lot of strong flavors to shine. This recipe delivers, thanks to a blend of bright, fresh herbs and a heavy dose of flavorful berries.

FOR THE MILLET

1½ cups uncooked millet

3 cups (770 ml) water

FOR THE DRESSING

1 tablespoon fresh mint leaves, minced

2 tablespoons fresh parsley or basil, minced

3 tablespoons fresh thyme leaves, minced

3 tablespoons walnut, almond, avocado, or liquid coconut oil

2 tablespoons raspberry vinegar

Juice of 1 lemon

2 tablespoons honey

Salt and pepper, to taste

⅓ cup (50 g) blueberries

⅓ cup (40 g) raspberries

⅓ cup (40 g) yellow raspberries

⅓ cup (40 g) chopped nuts or sunflower seeds

2 cups (60 g) baby spinach

1. To prepare the millet, add 3 cups of salted water to a medium saucepot over high heat. When the water reaches a boil, add the millet, reduce the heat to low, and cover the saucepot. Cook for ten to fifteen minutes or until all the water is absorbed. Remove from the heat and allow the millet to completely cool.

2. To make the dressing, add the mint, parsley, thyme, oil, vinegar, lemon juice, honey, salt, and pepper to a blender and process until smooth.

3. Remove millet to a serving container. Pour dressing over millet and mix gently until combined.

4. Gently fold in the berries, nuts, and spinach, being careful not to break berries.

5. Cover and let sit at room temperature for twenty minutes to allow the flavors to blend.

CURRIED CRANBERRY BARLEY

MAKES 6 SERVINGS

Barley is a chewy grain that is rich in protein, iron, vitamin B6, and magnesium. It makes a healthy, high-fiber side dish that goes with a variety of vegetarian, poultry, and meat dishes. This particular dish is flavored with curry, garlic, and cranberries.

1   tablespoon extra-virgin olive oil

1   cup (160 g) onions, diced

2   to 3 large garlic cloves, finely minced

1½ teaspoons mild curry powder

Salt and pepper, to taste

3   cups (700 ml) fat-free chicken broth

1½ cups (300 g) quick-cooking barley

1   cup (100 g) frozen cranberries

1   cup (145 g) raisins or dried cranberries

1   cup (100 g) pecans, chopped

1. Heat the oil in a large skillet over medium-high heat. Add the onions and sauté until barely tender, about four minutes.

2. Add the garlic and cook until onion is crisp-tender, about two additional minutes.

3. Stir in the curry, salt, pepper, and chicken broth.

4. Bring to a rolling boil and add the barley, cranberries, and raisins.

5. Reduce heat to low, cover, and simmer for fifteen to twenty minutes, or until all liquid is absorbed.

6. Remove from heat and allow mixture to cool slightly before stirring in the pecans.

VEGGIE SIDES

BLACKBERRY GREEN BEANS

MAKES 4 SERVINGS.

Versions of this recipe have been floating around the Internet for years. When I finally tried it, I was very pleasantly surprised by how well the ingredients work together. Feel free to add a few new potatoes if you'd like something more substantial. You can also make this recipe with asparagus spears, cut into 2-inch (5 cm) lengths, if desired, instead of green beans.

1   pound (55 g) green beans, trimmed

3   tablespoons extra-virgin olive oil, divided

1   medium-large yellow onion, halved and
    sliced into thin half-moons

1   tablespoon lemon juice

1½ tablespoons balsamic vinegar

1   teaspoon honey

½   cup (70 g) blackberries

Salt and pepper, to taste

1. In a medium-sized pot over high heat, bring salted water to a vigorous boil.

2. Add the green beans to the boiling water and cook for three minutes or until the beans are a vibrant green.

(continued)

3. Put the beans in a colander immediately, and run cold water over them to stop the cooking process. Leave the rinsed beans in the colander to dry while you get to the remaining steps.

4. Add 1 tablespoon olive oil to a large sauté pan over medium-low heat. Add the onions and cook, stirring very infrequently, about twenty minutes, or until they become a deep golden brown color. This process is called carmelization and it will take quite a while, so don't rush the process! (Fortunately, you don't need to do much with the onions as they carmelize.) Remove from the heat and set aside.

5. In a large bowl, whisk together lemon juice, balsamic vinegar, and 2 tablespoons olive oil, until emulsified. Add honey, salt, and pepper.

6. Add green beans and caramelized onions to the dressing and toss to coat.

7. Gently add berries, folding them in carefully so as to not break them.

8. Allow to sit, covered, at room temperature for thirty minutes for flavors to blend. Adjust vinegar, salt, and pepper before serving.

MASHED SWEET POTATOES WITH BERRIES

SERVES 4

This is a deeply nourishing, satisfying recipe and a delicious take on standard mashed sweet potatoes. The cranberries add a welcome tart note (plus vitamin C) to this earthy dish.

1 cup (50 g) walnuts or pecans

2 large sweet potatoes, peeled and sliced (about 1 pound/455 g each)

Salt and pepper, to taste

2 tablespoons roasted sesame oil or liquid coconut oil

2 tablespoons water, apple juice, or orange juice

2 tablespoons maple syrup

½ inch fresh ginger, minced

½ cup (50 g) dried unsweetened cranberries

1. Toast the nuts in a skillet over medium-high heat for about five minutes or until fragrant. Transfer them to a cutting board and chop.

2. Bring a saucepot full of salted water to a boil over high heat. Cook the sweet potatoes in the boiling water for about ten minutes or until soft. Drain, reserving ¼ cup (50 ml) cooking water. Transfer the sweet potatoes to a large bowl, and mash with reserved liquid. Season with salt and pepper.

3. Add the oil, water, maple syrup, ginger, and cranberries to a medium saucepot over medium-low heat and cook for two to five minutes or until fragrant and the cranberries begin to soften.

4. Add the cranberry mixture to the potatoes. Season with salt and pepper.

5. Serve sprinkled with the walnuts.

GOJI SPAGHETTI SQUASH

MAKES 4 SERVINGS

If you haven't tried spaghetti squash yet, you're in for a treat. The meat contains high levels of beta-carotene—for great skin and healthy eyesight. Here, spaghetti squash is made even healthier with immunity-boosting hydrated goji berries. This is a great Thanksgiving side dish!

3 large (about 3 pounds/1.35 kg each) spaghetti squash, halved lengthwise and seeds scraped

¼ cup (50 ml) extra-virgin olive oil, plus more for drizzling

Salt and freshly ground pepper, to taste

1 teaspoon chopped thyme

1 cup (250 ml) water

½ cup (125 ml) chicken or vegetable broth or dry white wine

¼ cup (28 g) hydrated goji berries

1. Preheat oven to 350°F (175°C or gas mark 4).

2. Place the spaghetti squash halves, cut sides up, on two large rimmed baking sheets. Rub the surface of each squash half with extra-virgin olive oil and season with salt, pepper, and thyme. Flip the squash cut sides down onto the baking sheets and pour the water and chicken broth into the pans. Bake for about fifty minutes, until the squash is barely tender.

3. Flip the cooked squash cut sides up and let them cool until warm.

4. Working over a large bowl, using a fork, scrape out the spaghetti squash, separating the strands. Add the remaining olive oil and goji berries to the bowl and toss to combine. Adjust seasonings before serving.

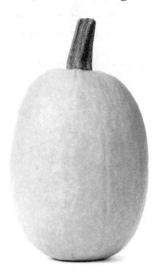

SPICY BERRY GREENS

MAKES 6 SERVINGS

This recipe is a blueprint of sorts for just about any greens you may have on hand. Collards, chard, tatsoi, and turnip greens are particularly delicious, but don't hold back—experiment with other greens too!

¼ cup (50 ml) liquid coconut oil or extra-virgin olive oil

3 to 5 garlic cloves, minced

3 bunches greens (either a single kind or a mix of greens), cleaned and thick stems and ribs removed)

Pinch of cayenne pepper

Salt and pepper, to taste

¾ cup (75 g) toasted walnuts or pecans, roughly chopped

⅓ cup (40 g) dried blueberries, unsweetened cranberries, or dried goji berries

Optional: 3 tablespoons to ¼ cup (50 ml) red wine vinegar for seasoning

1. Add the oil to a large pot over medium heat. Add the garlic and cook just until barely softened. Add about half the greens and toss with tongs.

2. Add the salt, pepper, cayenne pepper, and remaining greens to the pot, tossing to distribute.

3. Continue cooking, tossing often, until the excess liquid evaporates and the greens begin to soften. (This time may vary depending upon the greens you use.)

4. Add the walnuts and berries and toss gently.

5. Season with vinegar if desired and adjust salt and pepper before serving.

ELDERBERRIES: DID YOU KNOW?

- In Russia and England, elderberry trees were thought to ward off evil spirits, in years past, and it was considered good luck to plant an elderberry tree near one's home.

- In Sicily, sticks of elderberry wood were once thought to kill serpents and drive away thieves.

- In the Middle Ages throughout Europe, legend held that the elderberry tree was a home to witches and that cutting one down one would incur the wrath of any witch residing in the branches. It was believed that the only way to safely cut down an elderberry tree was to chant a rhyme to the "Elder Mother."

BRUSSELS SPROUTS WITH WALNUTS & DRIED CRANBERRIES

SERVES 6

I have to admit that the first time I tried Brussels sprouts I was not impressed. They were overcooked, simultaneously mealy and mushy, and incredibly smelly. Fortunately, I've had skillfully prepared sprouts since that time and truly love these super disease-fighting veggies. Here, they are dressed up with sweet-tart dried cranberries. Yum!

3   tablepoons walnut oil or extra-virgin olive oil, divided

1½ pounds (680 g) Brussels sprouts, halved

2   shallots, halved and sliced

1   clove garlic, minced

¼   cup (30 g) coarsely chopped dried unsweetened cranberries

1   tablespoon Grade B maple syrup

1   cup water

½   cup (60 g) coarsely chopped walnuts or pecans, toasted

Salt and pepper, to taste

1. Heat 2 tablespoons of the walnut oil in a large skillet over high heat. Add the Brussels sprouts and cook, stirring only occasionally, for four to five minutes until browned.

GOOSEBERRY & PAPAYA FACE PACK

MAKES ½ CUP

This is an incredible exfoliating mask, thanks to enzyme-rich papaya and gooseberry. But if your skin is sensitive, you might want to skip this one. You can buy rosewater in the baking section of some grocery stores, or at a store that specializes in Middle Eastern products.

¼   cup chopped papaya

¼   cup (25 g) gooseberries

2   tablespoons rosewater

1. Add all the ingredients to a food processor and pulse into a thick paste.

2. Use immediately. Start with clean skin and gently massage mixture onto the face, neck, and décolleté. Remove with cool water.

---

2. Add the shallots and garlic to the skillet and cook one minute.

3. Lower heat to medium and stir in the cranberries, maple syrup, and water. Partially cover the skillet, reduce the heat to medium, and simmer five to seven minutes or until most of the liquid has evaporated and Brussels sprouts are just fork tender.

4. Transfer the Brussels sprouts to a serving bowl and gently fold in the toasted walnuts, the rest of the walnut oil, salt, and pepper.

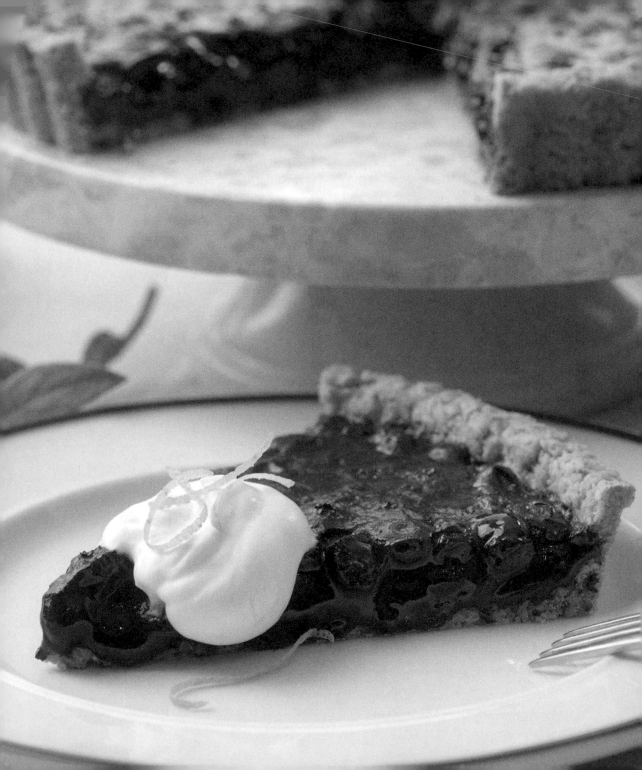

CHAPTER 8

BERRIES FOR DESSERT

Berry, berry, berry. I don't know about you, but the very word makes me think of dessert. From strawberry shortcake to blueberry tart to flourless chocolate cake with raspberry coulis, berries are the quintessential ending to a meal. But—you knew this was coming, didn't you?—too many berry recipes are loaded with sugar, butter, cream, white flour, and on and on, turning a health-supportive superfood into a health-damaging nightmare. What I'd like to do in this chapter is show you a different way to enjoy berry desserts. I promise that every recipe here is delicious—after all, what's the point of eating dessert if it doesn't taste fantastic? But these recipes are also good for you. Based on superfood ingredients, these treats make the most of berries' big, bold taste and their ability to improve your health. Enjoy!

DESSERT SOUPS & SALADS

BALSAMIC BERRIES

MAKES 4 SERVINGS

This is probably the most sophisticated recipe in the book, and, as you'll see, it's also the easiest. Balsamic berries are elegant and perfect as-is, but feel free to accessorize with a bit of cream or the lovely Whipped Coconut Cream (see page 150).

Juice and zest of 1 lemon

¼ cup (50 ml) balsamic vinegar

2 cups (330 g) sliced strawberries

2 cups (295 g) blueberries, blackberries, or mulberries

1 cup (125 g) raspberries

1. In a large bowl, whisk together the lemon juice, lemon zest, and vinegar.

2. Add the berries and very gently combine.

3. Cover and chill thirty minutes before serving.

OPPOSITE: **Blueberry Tart, page 152**

SMOOTH BERRY SOUP

MAKES 4 SERVINGS

I grew up eating fruit soup, so the idea of berry-based dessert soups is one that is very familiar to me. This beautiful raw soup features a blend of your favorite fresh or frozen berries. It also makes a nice brunch dish and a lovely snack.

- ¾ cup (85 g) black currants or blackberries
- ¾ cup (110 g) blueberries
- ¾ cup (85 g) red currants or raspberries
- ¾ cup (110 g) strawberries
- ¼ cup (80 ml) plus 2 tablespoons fresh-squeezed lime juice
- ½ tablespoon grated fresh ginger
- 1 teaspoon balsamic vinegar

1. Place all the ingredients in a blender or food processor and process until smooth.

2. Pour the mixture through a strainer or cheesecloth to catch all the seeds and pulp.

3. Place the soup in a tightly covered container and chill for three hours or overnight before serving.

CREAMY TREATS

BERRY CRÈME PARFAIT

MAKES 4 SERVINGS

Your family will love this easy, fun recipe. If you want to change things up, you can make individual trifles by adding crushed (healthy) cookies or cake between the berry and cream layers.

- 4 cups (515 g) raspberries, divided
- 1 cup (145 g) blackberries (or raspberries)
- 1 recipe Whipped Coconut Cream, divided (See page 150)

1. In a food processor or blender, process 1½ cups (185 g) raspberries until chunky. Or place the raspberries in a bowl and mash with the back of a fork or a potato masher.

2. In a large bowl, combine the mashed raspberries and 1 cup Whipped Coconut Cream.

3. Divide the mixture between four glass parfait cups or other containers.

4. Top the cups with more Whipped Coconut Cream.

5. Divide the rest of the raspberries among the parfait cups, placing berries directly on top of the dessert cream. Serve immediately.

BLUEBERRY FLUFF

MAKES 6 SERVINGS

Mmmmm . . . this is absolutely scrumptious. It's hard to believe something so yummy has only six ingredients! Blackberries or raspberries also work well in the berry fluff.

- *1 cup (150 g) raw cashews*
- *½ cup (125 ml) coconut milk (Do not use light.)*
- *3 tablespoons liquid coconut oil*
- *1 tablespoon coconut nectar or Grade B maple syrup*
- *1 teaspoon vanilla extract*
- *2 cups (310 g) frozen blueberries*

1. Place the cashews, coconut milk, coconut oil, coconut nectar, and vanilla extract in a blender or food processor and process until smooth.

2. Add the berries and process again until smooth and fluffy.

3. Serve immediately.

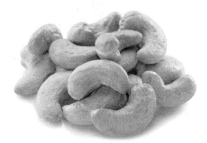

BERRY AVOCADO PUDDING

MAKES 4 SERVINGS

Those of you who have experimented with raw foods may know the avocado pudding trick, where you use a ripe avocado as the base for a creamy pudding, and then flavor it with chocolate or other ingredients. This is one of those puddings—made extra delicious with berries.

- *1 cup (147 g) chopped Medjool dates*
- *1 medium or large ripe Hass avocado, pitted, peeled, and chopped*
- *2 teaspoons lemon juice*
- *1 cup (125 g) fresh or frozen berries (raspberries, preferably)*
- *2 teaspoons vanilla extract*

Pinch of salt

1. Place the dates in a small bowl and add just enough warm water to cover them. Soak the dates for thirty minutes. Then thoroughly drain off the liquid. (You can save it to sweeten a smoothie!)

2. Place dates and all the remaining ingredients in a food processor or high-power blender and process until smooth.

3. Spoon into serving cups and enjoy immediately. Or chill before serving, if preferred.

CHOCOLATE-BERRY POTS DE CRÈME

MAKES 4 SERVINGS

Here, I pair chocolate with raspberries, but these berry pots de crème taste just as great with blackberries or black currants. While you won't taste it, coconut milk gives this recipe its creamy texture and heart-healthy, medium-chain fatty acids.

- 2 eggs
- ¼ (50 ml) cup honey
- 2 teaspoons vanilla extract
- ¾ cup (175 ml) coconut milk
- 1 cup (125 g) raspberries, blackberries, or black currants (plus a few more for garnish if desired)
- 4 ounces (115 g) chopped unsweetened chocolate

1. Add the eggs, honey, and vanilla to a food processor or blender and process until smooth.

2. In a small saucepot over high heat, warm the coconut milk until almost boiling.

3. As the coconut milk is heating, add the berries and chocolate to the egg-honey mixture in the blender and pulse until the ingredients become a paste.

4. When the coconut milk is very hot, slowly add it to the ingredients in the food processor or blender, processing on a low speed until chocolate is completely melted (the heat from the hot coconut milk will melt the chocolate) and the mixture is smooth and thick.

5. Pour the pudding into four ramekins or other serving containers and chill for two or more hours before serving. If desired, garnish with berries.

COCONUT MILK DEMYSTIFIED

Coconut milk is a delicious milky beverage that is created when mature coconut milk (either dried or not) is mixed with water. An essential ingredient in Pacific Island, Southeast Asian, West Indian, and Indian cooking, it has become a staple in health-conscious North American and European kitchens as well, where it is becoming a common replacement for dairy-based milk.

Canned coconut milk is still the most popular option around. But there are other excellent options, including frozen coconut milk, coconut milk beverage boxes and cartons (these are typically thinned with water and treated with various emulsifiers, flavorings, and stabilizers), and dried coconut milk that can be mixed with water.

COOKIES

ALMOND-BERRY SHORTBREAD

MAKES 15 COOKIES

This decadent cookie is a protein-rich way to enjoy dried unsweetened cranberries. You can also use dried blueberries if you can find them. I'm not crazy about using confectioners' sugar in this recipe, but I've tried other sweeteners with poor results. If you are absolutely opposed to using confectioners' sugar, whir 3 tablespoons of coconut sugar into a powder in a spice or coffee grinder and use that instead.

- *1 cup (110 g) almond flour*
- *3 tablespoons liquid coconut oil*
- *3 tablespoons confectioners' sugar*
- *⅛ teaspoon salt*
- *½ teaspoon vanilla extract*
- *½ teaspoon orange zest*
- *¼ cup (30 g) dried unsweetened cranberries*

1. In a stand mixer, add the almond flour, coconut oil, confectioners' sugar, salt, and vanilla. Mix on a low speed for two minutes or until just combined.

2. Add the orange zest and dried cranberries and mix just until combined.

3. Spoon the dough onto a large rectangle of wax paper or plastic wrap. Fashion into a roll about 7 inches (18 cm) long and 2 inches (5 cm) wide. Freeze for twenty minutes to chill.

4. Preheat oven to 350°F (175°C or gas mark 4).

5. Line a baking sheet with parchment paper or foil.

6. Remove the dough from the freezer and slice into ¼-inch (6-mm) cookies, placing each on the prepared sheet.

7. Bake for twelve minutes or until just firm to the touch and barely golden.

8. Cool on baking sheet for ten minutes before transferring to a cooling rack.

9. Place uneaten cookies in a tightly covered container and store for up to five days.

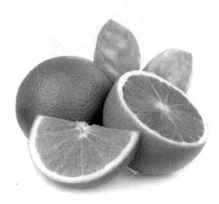

BLUEBERRY BREAKFAST COOKIES

MAKES 9 COOKIES

This is a rustic, bumpy, down-home kind of cookie filled with fruit and oats. It makes a great lunchbox treat and can even be included on a brunch menu—it's that good.

1   cup (225 g) mashed ripe bananas

½   cup (125 ml) pear sauce or applesauce

½   teaspoon vanilla extract

1½ cups (235 g) old-fashioned oats

½   teaspoon ground cinnamon

⅛   teaspoon salt

½   cup (75 g) fresh or frozen blueberries

1. Preheat oven to 350°F (175°C or gas mark 4).

2. Line a baking sheet with parchment paper or foil.

3. Whisk together the mashed bananas, pear sauce, and vanilla in a large bowl.

4. Stir in the oats, cinnamon, salt, and berries, mixing thoroughly to make a dough.

5. Drop tablespoons of the dough on the baking sheet and bake for twenty minutes or until cookies are light golden brown and slightly firm to the touch.

6. Cool the cookies before serving.

FLOURLESS PB&B COOKIES

MAKES ABOUT 18 COOKIES

This is my family's go-to cookie recipe. We make it with peanut butter, almond butter, cashew butter, or sunflower butter. Sometimes we add chocolate or dried fruit. You can dress them up even more by adding a dash of ground cinnamon, allspice, or ginger to the dough.

1   cup (260 g) natural peanut butter (Avoid runny natural peanut butter— you want a brand that has the same consistency as "regular" peanut butter.)

1   cup (220 g) packed golden brown sugar or coconut sugar

1   large egg

1   teaspoon baking soda

½   teaspoon vanilla extract

1   cup (150 g) fresh or frozen blueberries, hydrated goji berries, or dried unsweetened cranberries

1. Preheat oven to 350°F (175°C or gas mark 4).

2. Line two baking sheets with parchment paper or foil.

3. Combine the peanut butter, sugar (if using coconut sugar, whir in a coffee grinder first to create a finer-textured sugar), egg, baking soda, and vanilla extract, mixing until smooth.

4. Carefully stir in the berries, trying not to smash them.

5. With moistened hands, form generous balls of dough, about one tablespoon of dough for each cookie.

6. Space the cookies two inches apart on baking sheets.

7. Bake the cookies until puffed, golden on the bottom, and still soft to the touch in the center, about twelve minutes.

8. Cool the cookies on the baking sheets for about five minutes before serving.

BLUEBERRY TURMERIC ACNE MASK

MAKES ½ CUP

The blueberries in this mask help slough off dead skin cells and remove impurities from pores, while turmeric and lemon kill bacteria and encourage skin to heal.

- *¼ cup (25 g) blueberries*
- *2 teaspoons lemon juice*
- *½ teaspoon turmeric powder*

1. Add all the ingredients to a food processor and pulse into a thick paste.

2. Use immediately. Start with clean skin and gently massage mixture onto the face, neck, and décolleté. Leave on for 15 minutes before removing with cool water.

CAKES & SHORTCAKES

BERRY SHORTCAKE BISCUITS

MAKES 6 SHORTCAKES

This health-supportive shortcake recipe is based on almond flour, which offers up fiber, protein, calcium, iron, and magnesium. There are other nutritious ingredients, too, including coconut oil and berries!

- *2½ cups (140 g) almond flour*
- *½ teaspoon baking soda*
- *¼ teaspoon salt*
- *¼ cup (50 ml) liquid coconut oil*
- *1 tablespoon honey or coconut nectar*
- *2 large eggs*
- *¼ teaspoon vanilla extract*
- *1 teaspoon lemon or lime juice*
- *1 tablespoon honey*
- *2 cups (290 g) strawberries or another berry*
- *Optional: Whipped Coconut Cream (see page 150)*

1. In a small bowl, whisk together the almond flour, baking soda, and salt. Set aside.

2. In a medium bowl, whisk together the coconut oil and honey until smooth.

(continued)

3. Add the eggs and vanilla to the oil-honey mixture and whisk until thoroughly combined.

4. Add the almond flour mixture to the wet ingredients and stir until thoroughly combined.

5. Cover the bowl and chill for twenty minutes to firm up.

6. Preheat oven to 350°F (175°C or gas mark 4).

7. Line a baking sheet with parchment paper; set aside.

8. While the dough is chilling, whisk together the lemon juice and honey in a large bowl.

9. Add the berries and gently stir to coat. Cover the bowl and chill to allow flavors to meld.

10. Take out the dough and use a tablespoon, a cookie scoop, or your hands to make balls of dough the size of Ping-Pong balls. Place these on the prepared baking sheet, lightly flattening each with the palm of your hand or the bottom of a heavy tumbler.

11. Bake the biscuits for about fifteen minutes, until golden brown on top and a toothpick inserted into the center comes out clean.

12. Split the warm biscuits in half and top with a couple heaping spoonfuls of the strawberry topping and if desired, a spoonful of Whipped Coconut Cream (below).

WHIPPED COCONUT CREAM

Are you looking for a luscious alternative to whipped cream? Look no further! There's one for you right here, and it harnesses all the heath-supportive benefits of coconut!

TO MAKE THE TOPPING: Grab a 14-ounce (414 ml) can of coconut cream (do not use sweetened cream of coconut) and shake it well. Leave the can in the refrigerator overnight, then remove it and shake it well again. Empty the contents into the bowl of a stand mixer, add 1 tablespoon of vanilla extract (or 1 to 2 teaspoons of your favorite liquor), and spoon in 1 to 3 tablespoons powdered sugar. Using the whisk attachment of the mixer, begin to beat the coconut cream and slowly increase the speed to medium. Beat the mixture until the coconut cream looks light and airy, about three to five minutes. Use this delicious stuff whenever and wherever you'd normally use whipped dairy cream.

CHOCOLATE-BERRY TORTE

MAKES 10 SERVINGS

Every cook needs a good flourless chocolate cake! This one, because it's based on ground nuts (walnuts or pecans), qualifies as a "torte." It is a gorgeous dinner-party dessert that will impress anyone who tries it. The recipe contains cane sugar, however—a bit more than I wish, to be truthful, but I just haven't found another way for this recipe to work without it. Just promise me you'll stop at one slice and all will be well!

¾ cup (110 g) firm blackberries or raspberries

½ cup (125 ml) liquid coconut oil, plus extra for oiling the pan

8 ounces (225 g) bittersweet chocolate, chopped

1¼ cups (250 g) natural cane sugar

4 large eggs

¼ cup (20 g) unsweetened cocoa powder, plus ½ tablespoon for dusting the cake pan

1 teaspoon vanilla extract

½ teaspoon coarse salt

½ cup (40 g) ground toasted walnuts or pecans

1. Preheat oven to 350°F (175°C or gas mark 4).

2. Lightly oil an 8-inch (20-cm) round cake pan and line the bottom of the pan with parchment paper. Oil the parchment and then dust the entire inside of the cake pan with the ½ tablespoon cocoa powder.

3. Scatter the berries in the bottom of the prepared pan. Set aside.

4. In a double boiler, combine ½ cup (125 ml) of the oil and the bittersweet chocolate, stirring until the chocolate is melted and the mixture is smooth.

5. Remove from the heat and whisk in the sugar.

6. Next, whisk in the eggs, one at a time, followed by ¼ cup (20 g) of cocoa powder, vanilla, and salt.

7. Gently fold in the nuts.

8. Spread the batter in the pan.

9. Bake until set, about thirty-five minutes. Let the torte cool completely in the pan, preferably overnight.

10. To remove the torte from the pan, run a knife around the edges to loosen.

11. Wrap uneaten torte in food wrap or place in a covered container and store in the fridge for up to three days.

PIES & TARTS

BLUEBERRY TART

MAKES 8 SERVINGS

This is a wonderful tart that just happens to be high in antioxidants and fiber. The nut-based crust adds protein, minerals, and additional fiber. *Note:* We like our fruit desserts less sweet than some people. You won't hurt my feelings if you add two more tablespoons of sweetener to the filling!

FOR THE CRUST

1⅓ cup (105 g) cold-fashioned oats

1   cup (240 g) walnuts

2   tablespoons sugar

⅛ teaspoon salt

1   egg

FOR THE FILLING

1½ pounds (680 g) fresh or frozen blueberries

½ cup (75 g) coconut sugar, honey, Grade B maple sugar, or light brown sugar

1½ tablespoons freshly squeezed lemon juice

1   teaspoon ground cinnamon

2   tablespoons arrowroot powder

2   tablespoons cold water

1. TO MAKE THE CRUST: Preheat oven to 350°F (175°C or gas mark 4).

2. Lightly oil a 10-inch (25-cm) tart pan. Set aside.

3. Combine the oats, walnuts, sugar, and salt in a food processor and pulse three or four times, or until chunky.

4. Add the egg and pulse until ingredients are thoroughly combined.

5. With moistened fingertips, press dough evenly into the tart pan. Poke the crust in several places with a fork and bake for twelve minutes, or until lightly browned.

6. Allow the crust to cool while you make the fruit filling.

7. TO MAKE THE FILLING: Add blueberries to a small saucepot over medium heat. Bring to a boil and then reduce the heat to medium-low. Allow berries to gently simmer for about eight minutes or until they begin to get soft.

8. Add the sugar, lemon juice, and cinnamon, and cook for another two minutes.

9. In a small bowl, whisk together the arrowroot powder and water, then stir the mixture into the simmering berry mixture.

10. Continue to cook the tart filling for another one to two minutes. Remove the filling from heat and cool for ten to fifteen minutes, or until it reaches room temperature.

11. Spoon the mixture into the tart crust and chill for at least two hours before serving.

KEY LIME-AVOCADO BERRY PIE

MAKES 8 SERVINGS

One look at the title of this recipe and you see it has a lot of superfood action going on. If you haven't used avocado in a dessert before, I invite you to try it right now! I think you'll be surprised at how easy it is to make this divine pie and how good it tastes.

FOR THE CRUST

2 cups (170 g) dried unsweetened coconut flakes (medium or fine shreds)

2½ tablespoons coconut oil, softened

1½ tablespoons coconut flour

Dash of salt

¼ cup honey or coconut nectar

2 teaspoons vanilla extract

Optional: Zest from 1 or 2 limes or key limes

FOR THE FILLING

1½ (345 g) cups mashed Hass avocado (about 2 large avocados)

Zest from 1 or 2 limes or key limes

¾ cup (175 ml) lime or key lime juice

½ cup (125 ml) honey

Pinch of salt

½ cup (125 ml) liquid coconut oil, plus extra for oiling the pan

1½ cups (185 g) raspberries

1. TO MAKE THE CRUST: Preheat oven to 350°F (175°C or gas mark 4).

2. Lightly oil an 8-inch (20-cm) pie pan.

3. Add the coconut flakes, coconut oil, coconut flour, salt, honey, vanilla, and lime zest (optional) to the bowl of a stand mixer. Mix until a sticky dough appears, adding 1 to 3 teaspoons of additional honey if needed to create a cohesive, sticky mass.

4. With moistened fingers, pat the piecrust mixture into the prepared pie pan and bake for eight to ten minutes, or until edges start to turn a golden brown.

5. Very gently remove the piecrust from the oven and place it on the counter to cool. It is very fragile and crumbly until it cools and "sets up." Allow the crust to cool for twenty minutes before transferring it to the freezer to harden further.

6. TO MAKE THE FILLING: Add the avocados, lime zest, lime juice, honey, salt, and coconut oil in a food processor and process until completely smooth.

7. Add the berries to the processor and pulse three or four times to just break up some of the berries. You want to keep some of them whole.

8. Transfer the avocado-berry mixture to the now-frozen piecrust and freeze the pie for one additional hour to firm up.

CRISPS & COBBLERS & MORE

BERRY SLUMP

MAKES 6 SERVINGS

A slump is a cobbler that you cook on the stovetop, rather than bake in the oven. This rustic-looking dessert is easy to make, delicious, and versatile. Feel free to use a different sweetener or other berries, and sneak in some ginger or cinnamon or lemon—or something else entirely; this recipe is eminently customizable!

3   cups (430 g) blackberries

¾   cup (110 g) water or unsweetened cranberry juice

¾   cup (175 g) coconut sugar or regular sugar, divided

¾   cup (95 g) all-purpose flour or gluten-free flour

1   teaspoon baking powder

1   teaspoon ground cinnamon

⅛   teaspoon salt

3   tablespoons solid coconut oil, cold

⅓   cup (80 ml) coconut milk or nut milk

1. Combine the berries, water, and ½ cup (115 g) of the sugar in a large saucepot over medium-high heat. Bring the mixture to a boil, reduce the heat to low, and simmer until liquid thickens to a syrupy consistency, about twenty minutes.

2. In a medium bowl, stir together the flour, the remaining ¼ cup (55 g) of sugar, baking powder, cinnamon, and salt.

3. Add the solid coconut oil by cutting it into the flour mixture and working it into the dry ingredients with two forks or a handheld pastry blender until the mixture resembles crumbs.

4. Add the coconut milk to the flour mixture and stir just until lightly mixed. Be careful not to overmix.

5. Spoon small mounds of the dough on top of the simmering fruit mixture to create dumplings. (It will "slump" together to cover the mixture.) Simmer covered until a toothpick inserted into the dumplings comes out clean, after about fifteen to twenty minutes.
Note: Dumplings will cook through but remain soft in texture.

6. Serve warm.

BLUEBERRY CRISP

MAKES 6 SERVINGS

Crisps are among the easiest baked desserts to make. Simply choose a fruit, dump it in a baking pan, and sprinkle it with a quickly made topping. The blueberries, almonds, and pecans in this recipe make for a yummy dish that is also high in protein, fiber, and antioxidants.

Note: The fruit in this dessert is unsweetened. Feel free to stir a couple tablespoons of honey into the berries before placing them in the baking pan. Also, blueberries—and cranberries, too—have plenty of pectin to naturally thicken the filling. If you go with another berry, however, gently stir 2 teaspoons of arrowroot into your berries before placing them in the baking pan.

> 2 pints (295 g) blueberries
> 1½ cups (165 g) almond flour
> 1 cup (110 g) chopped pecans
> ¼ teaspoon sea salt
> ¼ cup (50 ml) liquid coconut oil
> ¼ cup (50 ml) coconut nectar, honey, or Grade B maple syrup

1. Preheat oven to 350°F (175°C or gas mark 4).

2. Grease a 9 × 11-inch (23 × 28-cm) baking pan.

3. Place the blueberries in the baking pan.

4. In a large bowl, combine the almond flour, pecans, salt, coconut oil, and coconut nectar until crumbly. Scatter the mixture across the blueberries.

5. Bake the crumble for forty-five to fifty minutes or until the fruit is bubbling and the topping is golden brown. If the topping browns too quickly, cover loosely with foil.

RASPBERRY WRINKLE SOFTENER

MAKES ABOUT 3 TABLESPOONS

This lovely mask is a bit messy, but it's very effective. It softens, smoothes, plumps, firms, and moisturizes the skin.

> 1 tablespoon almond oil
> 2 tablespoons dry oatmeal, ground into a powder
> 8 raspberries

1. In a bowl, whisk together the oil and ground oats until smooth.

2. Add the raspberries, mashing them into the mixture with the back of a fork. Mix until combined.

3. Use immediately. Start with clean skin and gently massage mixture onto the face, neck, and décolleté. Leave on for 20 before removing with cool water.

RED COBBLER

MAKES 4 SERVINGS

A cobbler is like a crisp, but with a different kind of topping. Spoonfuls of dough are dropped onto and then smoothed over the filling to create a more crust-like surface. This cobbler boasts strawberries and raspberries for a high-antioxidant dish that is as nourishing as it is delicious. Feel free to try different berry combinations.

FOR THE FILLING

2   cups (290 g) strawberries, halved

2   cups (245 g) raspberries

2   tablespoons tapioca starch

2   teaspoons vanilla extract

1   tablespoon lemon juice

1   tablespoon Grade B maple syrup

FOR THE TOPPING

1   cup (110 g) almond flour

½   teaspoon salt

3   tablespoons liquid coconut oil

3   tablespoons Grade B maple syrup

1. Preheat oven to 350°F (175°C or gas mark 4).

2. In a large bowl, combine the strawberries, raspberries, tapioca starch, vanilla, lemon juice, and maple syrup.

3. Pour the mixture into an 8-inch (20-cm) square baking pan. Set aside.

4. In a large bowl, mix together the almond flour, salt, coconut oil, and maple syrup.

5. Using a tablespoon, drop spoonfuls of the topping over the fruit mixture. Using an offset spatula, smooth the dough over the top of the fruit mixture.

6. Bake for thirty minutes, or until the strawberries are juicy and bubbly and the topping is golden brown.

7. Let stand for ten minutes before serving.

MULBERRY FACE PACK

MAKES 3 TABLESPOONS

This easy-to-make mask features just two ingredients: Mulberries and coconut milk. It strengthens and firms the skin. You'll love it!

5   mulberries

2   tablespoons coconut milk (not light)

1. In a bowl, smash the mulberries into a paste using the back of a fork.

2. Whisk in the coconut milk until blended.

3. Use immediately. Start with clean skin and gently massage mixture onto the face, neck, and décolleté. Leave on for 15 minutes before removing with cool water.

FROZEN DESSERTS

BERRY SORBET

MAKES 4 SERVINGS

Sorbet is ice cream's healthier, more sophisticated cousin. Commercially made sorbets, however, and even recipes for homemade sorbet, contain outrageous amounts of corn syrup and processed sugar. This more health-supportive recipe for berry sorbet uses sweeteners that have a lower glycemic index and some nutritive value. (It won't get as icy-hard as store-bought sorbet, though.) Feel free to use whatever berries or blends of berries (and other fruit), you'd like.

Note: You'll need an ice cream maker for this one.

1½ cups (350 ml) unsweetened cranberry (or other berry) juice or water

½ cup (125 ml) maple syrup, honey, or coconut sugar

3 cups (370 g) berries (one type or a blend of mulberries, red or black currants, strawberries, raspberries, blueberries, or blackberries)

3 tablespoons lemon or lime juice

1. Combine the juice and maple syrup in a heavy saucepot over medium-high heat and bring to a boil. Cook, stirring occasionally, until the syrup is completely dissolved.

2. Add the berries and return to a boil. Lower the heat to medium-low and simmer, stirring constantly, until the berries are soft and beginning to lose their shape.

3. Strain the berries through a fine-mesh sieve into a bowl, pressing on the berries with the back of a large spoon. Discard the pulp and seeds. Alternately, you could blend the mixture in a food processor or high-powered blender until very, very smooth.

4. Stir in the lemon juice.

5. Chill for two to three hours.

6. Pour the cooled mixture into an ice cream maker and freeze according to the manufacturer's directions.

7. When finished, transfer the sorbet to a tightly covered container and freeze for two to three hours until the sorbet is firm.

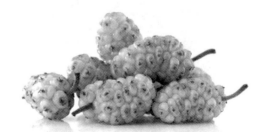

White mulberries

BERRY GRANITA

MAKES 4 SERVINGS

Granitas are like adult slushies—icy, sweet, and intensely flavored. They are also easy to make and a great way to preserve the health-giving benefits of berries.

Note: You do not need an ice cream maker for this recipe.

2   cups (245 g) berries, a single variety or a mix of types

2   tablespoons honey

1   tablespoon lemon or lime juice

1   cup (155 g) ice

1. Blend the berries, honey, lemon juice, and ice in a food processor or blender until smooth.

2. Pour the mixture into an 8-inch (20-cm) square baking pan. Freeze for thirty minutes.

3. Remove the baking pan from the freezer and rake the mixture with a fork until slushy.

4. Return the baking pan to the freezer for one hour or until set.

5. Freeze any uneaten granita in a covered container.

BERRY-AVOCADO ICE CREAM

MAKES 4 SERVINGS

Avocado ice cream? It does sounds strange, doesn't it? But I strongly encourage you to give it a try. It's amazing! Avocado provides brain-protective glutathione and heart-healthy fat, while berries add vitamin C, fiber, and antioxidants for a strong immune system and healthy skin.

Note: You'll need an ice cream maker for this recipe.

2½ cups (600 ml) full-fat coconut or nut milk (Use a brand with no stabilizers or sweeteners.)

2   large, ripe Hass avocados

1   cup (125 g) berries, either a single variety or a combination of varieties

½   cup (75 g) coconut sugar or regular sugar

1   tablespoon lemon or lime juice

Pinch of salt

1. Add all the ingredients to a food processor or blender and process until thoroughly blended and very smooth.

2. Pour the mixture into an ice cream maker and freeze according to the manufacturer's directions.

3. When finished, transfer the ice cream to a tightly covered container and freeze.

COULIS:
THE PERFECT DESSERT ACCESSORY

MIXED BERRY COULIS
MAKES ABOUT 2 CUPS (475 ML)

One of the easiest ways to upgrade any dessert is to drape it with a beautiful sauce. And one of the most sophisticated dessert sauces around is the coulis. The word itself comes from an old French word meaning "to strain." It originally referred to any sauce—vegetable, fruit, or meat— that was strained to a smooth, silky finish. Today, we tend to think of coulis as a silky berry sauce. While most modern recipes for coulis are based on raspberries, this one can be made with any blend of fresh or frozen berries.

- 3 cups (370 g) fresh or frozen mixed berries (blueberries, raspberries, mulberries, red currants, black currants, strawberries, blackberries, etc.)
- ¼ cup (55 g) honey, coconut sugar, or regular sugar
- ¼ cup (50 ml) water or unsweetened cranberry juice
- 1 tablespoon lemon juice
- ½ teaspoon arrowroot starch
- Optional: 1 tablespoon orange or berry liquor, crème de cassis, or black currant syrup

1. Combine the berries, honey, and water in a large saucepot. Bring to a simmer, stirring occasionally.

2. Mix the lemon juice and arrowroot starch; add to the berry mixture and cook, stirring, until slightly thickened, about one minute. Stir in the orange or berry liquor or black currant syrup if desired.

3. Cool to room temperature. Strain through cheesecloth, a sieve, or a colander before serving.

4. **MAKE AHEAD TIP:** Cover and chill for up to four days.

CANDY

CHOCOLATE-DIPPED STRAWBERRIES

MAKES 12 STRAWBERRIES

Chocolate-dipped strawberries are so romantic! And they're also healthy if you use a dark, naturally sweetened chocolate. These are a bit of a project, so make sure you have a clean space and a quiet hour to make them.

Note: In this recipe, the strawberries need to be completely dry. Use a hair dryer to direct cool air on them if you need to get rid of any moisture.

6.25 ounces (175 g) chopped dark chocolate (You can use dark chocolate chips.)

1 dozen large strawberries with stems

1. Line a baking sheet with parchment paper or foil.

2. Melt the chocolate, either in a double boiler or a microwave. (Use twenty-second intervals and stir after each one.)

3. Remove from double boiler or microwave.

4. Working quickly, place a toothpick through the top of each strawberry. Holding this toothpick, dip the berry into the chocolate.

5. Place the dipped berry on the prepared baking sheet. Repeat with remaining strawberries.

6. Place baking sheet in the refrigerator and allow chocolate to harden, about two hours.

7. Once all strawberries' chocolate has become firm, place baking sheet in freezer for about ten minutes to allow chocolate to set up. They will be finished once all the sheen is gone from the chocolate.

8. Place each strawberry in a mini muffin liner or candy cup and refrigerate for up to three days in a covered container.

BLUEBERRY CHOCOLATE CLUSTERS

MAKES 18 SERVINGS

These treats are a riff on the popular chocolate-dipped strawberry. They are delicious, easy, and fun to make. And they are so much healthier than mainstream chocolate candy.

Note: For this recipe, the blueberries need to be completely dry. Use a hair dryer to direct cool air on the berries if you need to get rid of any moisture.

1 cup (150 g) blueberries, divided

1 cup (175 g) chopped dark chocolate (You can use dark chocolate chips.)

1. Line a baking sheet with parchment paper or foil.

2. Melt the chocolate, either in a double boiler or a microwave. (Use twenty-second intervals and stir after each one.)

3. Remove from double boiler or microwave and gently fold in the blueberries.

4. Make clusters by spooning four or five chocolate-coated blueberries onto the baking sheet, placing them 1 inch (2.5 cm) apart.

5. Place the baking sheet in the refrigerator and allow the chocolate to harden, about two hours.

6. Place each cluster in a mini muffin liner or candy cup and refrigerate for up to three days in a covered container.

DARK CHOCOLATE SUPERFOOD BARK

MAKES ABOUT 8 SERVINGS

Dark chocolate has its own antioxidants, but add dried goji berries, cranberries, and seeds, and you get even more of these powerful anti-inflammatory and immunity-building ingredients—plus a good dose of fiber and protein.

20 ounces (565 g) dark chocolate, chopped (You can use dark chocolate chips.)

¼ cup dried goji berries

¼ cup dried unsweetened cranberries

¼ cup raw sunflower seeds, pepitas, or chopped nut of your choice

2 tablespoons chia seeds

1. Line a baking sheet with parchment paper or foil.

2. Melt the chocolate, either in a double boiler or a microwave. (Use twenty-second intervals and stir after each one.)

3. Pour the melted chocolate onto the parchment paper and, using a flat spatula, spread it in an even layer about ¼-inch (6-mm) thick.

4. Sprinkle the goji berries, cranberries, sunflower seeds, and chia over the layer of chocolate.

5. Place baking sheet in the refrigerator and allow the chocolate bark to harden, about two hours.

6. Break into chunks and refrigerate in an airtight container for up to two weeks.

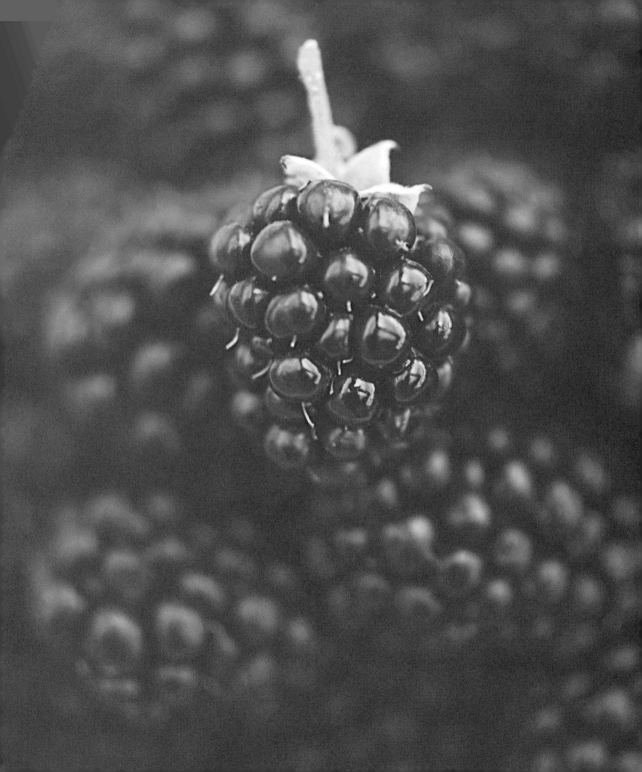

CHAPTER 9

BERRY CONDIMENTS

Berries make delicious, healthful condiments. The most famous of these—at least in North America—is cranberry sauce, which shows up on so many tables at Thanksgiving dinner every year. But berries are just as delicious tucked into a salsa, folded into avocado, whirred into hummus, or fashioned into a variety of marinades, sauces, and dressings. If you don't believe me, read this chapter. I promise it will make you see berries in a delicious new way!

SAUCES

SWEET & SOUR BLACK CURRANT SAUCE

MAKES 2 CUPS (475 ML)

This tangy British-style cooked sauce is a lovely marinade for game, pork, and poultry. It's also great drizzled over cooked meats or even used as a dressing for a green salad, grain salad, or roasted vegetables.

Note: Because broth plays such an important role in this sauce, please use the most delicious one you can find.

1 *cup (250 ml) good-quality chicken or vegetable broth*

1 *shallot, peeled and minced*

1 *teaspoon fresh thyme leaves*

3 *cups (335 g) black currants or elderberries*

1 *tablespoon honey*

½ *cup (125 ml) apple cider vinegar*

1 *teaspoon extra-virgin olive oil*

Salt and pepper, to taste

1. Add broth to a large saucepot over medium-high heat. When it boils, reduce heat to low and allow it to simmer until it appears to be reduced by half, about fifteen minutes.

2. Add the shallot and cook until soft.

3. Add the thyme leaves and currants, coating the currants with the chicken stock.

4. Add the honey and vinegar.

5. Simmer until the currants have become jammy, about seven to ten minutes.

(continued)

6. Remove from the heat and allow the sauce to cool slightly.

7. Pour the sauce into a food processor with the olive oil and process until smooth.

8. Taste the sauce and adjust with salt and pepper as needed.

MUSTARDS

BLACKBERRY MUSTARD

MAKES 1½ CUPS (350 ML)

This elegant mustard is dark and beautiful. It's healthy, too, thanks to the antioxidants contained in the blackberries. Try it with fresh raspberries, blueberries, or cranberries (even leftover cranberry sauce) if desired. This delicious mustard pairs well with poultry, pork, game, and cheeses. Try it on your next sandwich!

1 cup (145 g) blackberries
½ cup (125 ml) whole-grain mustard
½ to 1 tablespoon honey
Salt and pepper, to taste

1. Add all the ingredients to a food processor and process until smooth.

2. Refrigerate in a tightly covered container or jar for up to two weeks.

KETCHUPS

EASY CURRY-BERRY KETCHUP

MAKES 2½ CUPS (600 ML)

This fun, fruity, tangy ketchup is a surprising change from the regular variety. It's great with fries, burgers, hot dogs, and more.

2 cups (295 g) fresh or frozen blueberries
¼ cup (50 ml) honey
2 teaspoons curry powder (I like masala)
½ tablespoon water
1 cup (240 g) store-bought ketchup

1. Add the blueberries, honey, curry powder, and water to a medium saucepot over medium heat.

2. Bring them to a boil and simmer, stirring often just until the mixture is thick and sticky. Don't let mixture get so thick that you cannot move a spoon through it, however, as it will thicken naturally as it cools.

3. Take the mixture off the heat and cool. Don't be alarmed if it does thicken a bit once you remove the mixture from the heat.

4. Add the berry mixture and ketchup to a food processor and blend until smooth.

5. Refrigerate unused ketchup in a tightly covered container for up to two weeks.

SPICY BERRY KETCHUP

MAKES 1½ CUPS

Admittedly, this recipe has a lot going on. But it is so delicious and healthy (thanks to so many berries and chile and garlic and spices) that I urge you to give it a try.

1   *tablespoon extra-virgin olive oil*

1   *small yellow onion, chopped*

1   *jalapeno chile, seeded and chopped*

1   *garlic clove, chopped*

¾   *cup (110 g) blueberries*

¾   *cup (92 g) raspberries*

2   *tablespoons balsamic vinegar*

1   *tablespoon honey*

Salt and pepper, to taste

⅛   *teaspoon ground cinnamon*

⅛   *teaspoon ground ginger*

⅛   *teaspoon ground cloves*

⅛   *teaspoon ground allspice*

1. Heat the oil in small saucepot over medium-low heat. Add the onion and sauté, stirring often, until golden, about four minutes.

2. Add the jalapeno and garlic and cook until fragrant, about one minute.

3. Turn the heat up to medium and add remaining ingredients. Simmer until the mixture begins to thicken and bubble, about five minutes.

4. Remove from heat and allow the mixture to cool to room temperature.

5. Pour into a food processor and process until smooth.

6. Use immediately or refrigerate in an airtight container for up to two weeks.

STRAWBERRIES: DID YOU KNOW?

- Strawberries are the only fruit with seeds on the outside.

- The average strawberry has 200 seeds.

- About 94 percent of US households consume strawberries at least once a year.

- According to folklore, if a person cuts a strawberry in half to share, the two people consuming it together will fall in love. Maybe this is why they're believed to be an aphrodisiac in France, where strawberries, in the form of a creamy sweet soup, are served to newlyweds at traditional wedding breakfasts.

- To symbolize perfection and righteousness, medieval stonemasons carved strawberry designs on altars and around the tops of pillars in churches and cathedrals.

BARBECUE SAUCES

STRAWBERRY BARBECUE SAUCE

MAKES 2 CUPS (475 ML)

Several versions of this strawberry barbecue sauce exist. This one, however, is low in sugar. This barbecue sauce works well on poultry, beef, pork and even shrimp, vegetables, and roasted potatoes.

2⅓ cups (335 g) fresh or frozen and thawed strawberries

½ cup (125 ml) store-bought ketchup

¼ cup (50 ml) honey

3 tablespoons soy sauce

2 tablespoons lemon juice

2 tablespoons ground ginger

½ teaspoon hot sauce or ¼ teaspoon ground cayenne

Salt and pepper to taste

3 tablespoons green onions (scallions), chopped

1. Combine all the ingredients in a food processor and process until smooth.

2. Pour the sauce into a tightly covered container and store in the refrigerator for up to two weeks.

BLUEBERRY BARBECUE SAUCE

MAKES 3 CUPS (700 ML)

The deep, full-bodied, sweet, tangy taste makes this barbecue sauce a favorite. And as a nutritionist, I love all the antioxidants in this berry-rich sauce. I especially like it on pork, but it works just as well on poultry, beef, and even grilled corn on the cob, according to my kids!

2 cups (295 g) fresh or frozen blueberries

¾ cup (180 g) store-bought ketchup

½ cup (125 ml) apple cider vinegar

½ cup (175 g) coconut nectar or honey

1 teaspoon chili powder (especially one that contains chipotle)

Salt, to taste

1 teaspoon ground black pepper

½ cup (125 ml) unsweetened blueberry juice, unsweetened red currant, cranberry, or other berry juice, or water

1. In a large saucepot over medium heat, combine the blueberries, ketchup, vinegar, coconut sugar, chili powder, salt, and pepper.

2. Stir in the juice, increase heat to high, and bring the mixture to a boil, stirring to prevent sticking. Allow it to boil for about thirty seconds.

3. Reduce the heat to low and simmer, stirring occasionally, until the sauce has thickened.

4. Remove from the heat and allow the sauce to cool.

5. The sauce will be chunky. Use as-is, or (my preference) puree in a food processor or blender until smooth.

6. Store in a covered container in the refrigerator for up to two weeks.

CHUTNEYS, RELISHES & SALSAS

BLUEBERRY CHUTNEY

MAKES 1 CUP (250 ML)

This tangy chutney is lovely with pork and poultry or spooned on crackers, but I've also caught various people in my household enjoying it straight from the jar. Luckily, it's good for you, thanks to the onions, raisins, and blueberries, which, together, give you fiber, vitamins, and a host of cancer-fighting phytonutrients.

½   cup (80 g) chopped onion
¼   cup (35 g) coconut sugar or regular sugar or honey
1   ¼-inch (6-mm) slice of fresh ginger, minced
¼   cup (35 g) raisins
¼   cup (50 ml) apple cider vinegar
1   cup (150 g) blueberries, divided

1. Combine the onion, sugar, ginger, raisins, and vinegar in a small saucepot over medium-high heat and bring mixture to a boil.

2. Stir and reduce heat to medium-low. Simmer for three to five minutes, until the sugar has dissolved and onions are soft.

3. Continue simmering and add ½ cup (75 g) of the blueberries. Cook until jammy.

4. Add the remaining ½ cup (75 g) blueberries and simmer another two minutes or until berries begin to soften.

5. Allow the chutney to cool to room temperature. Refrigerate leftovers in a tightly covered container for up to five days.

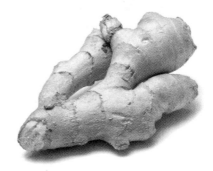

RED CURRANT & ROSEMARY CHUTNEY

MAKES 2½ CUPS (600 ML)

This sophisticated version of chutney, a truly international condiment, features red currants, which provide vitamins C and K, iron, protein, fiber, and a host of phytonutrients that help ward off cancer and strengthen the immune system. There is a fair amount of sweetener in this chutney, but feel free to use as much or as little of the sweetener as desired.

> 2½ cups (280 g) red currants
>
> 1½ cups (220 g) coconut sugar, honey, or other sweetener
>
> ½ cup (125 ml) red wine vinegar
>
> 1 large onion, finely chopped
>
> 1 small red bell pepper, finely chopped
>
> 1 garlic clove, minced or crushed
>
> 1 ¾- to 1-inch (10- to 25-mm) piece of fresh ginger, grated
>
> Dash of cayenne pepper
>
> 4 sprigs fresh rosemary, leaves removed and finely chopped

1. Add the red currants, sugar, and vinegar to a saucepot over medium heat.

2. Stir in the rest of the ingredients.

3. Bring the mixture to a boil, reducing heat to low, and allowing mixture to simmer for thirty minutes. Don't overcook: Though the chutney may look runny, it will firm up as it cools, thanks to the natural pectin in the currants.

4. Allow the chutney to cool to room temperature. Refrigerate leftovers in a tightly covered container for up to three days.

CRANBERRY RELISH

MAKES 3 CUPS (700 ML)

This is a no-cook "Thanksgiving-style" cranberry relish that can be used year-round as a salsa or side dish or to dress poultry and pork. In this recipe, tart cranberries get sweetness from apples and brightness from oranges.

> 1 crisp large apple of any variety, chopped
>
> 1 navel orange, peeled and chopped
>
> 2 cups (200 g) fresh cranberries (You can use frozen and thawed, but they will be softer), roughly chopped
>
> 1 cup (100 g) pecans, chopped
>
> ¼ cup (50 ml) honey, coconut sugar (55 g), or regular sugar (55 g)

1. Combine all the ingredients in a large bowl.

2. Refrigerate the leftovers in a covered container for up to three days.

MANGO GOJI AVOCADO SALSA

MAKES ABOUT 2 CUPS (475 ML)

The mango and dried goji berries in this delicious salsa provide antioxidants for a strong immune system, while the avocado offers healthy fats for brain, skin, and heart health.

> 1½ medium Hass avocados, diced
> 1   mango, diced
> 1½ tablespoons dried goji berries
> Juice of 2 limes or small lemons
> Salt and pepper, to taste

1. Place the avocado, mango, and goji berries in a large bowl. No need to combine.

2. Drizzle lime juice over the avocado-mango-goji berry mixture and sprinkle with salt and pepper. Very gently combine ingredients.

3. Use immediately.

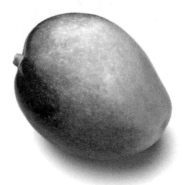

BLUEBERRY & TOMATO SALSA

MAKES 2¼ CUPS (525 ML)

This interesting recipe features traditional salsa ingredients—tomatoes, bell peppers, parsley, cilantro—along with the unusual addition of blueberries. Yes, it sounds weird. But it's so good! Do give it a try. For something different, replace the tomato with chopped pineapple and the vinegar with lime juice.

- 1 cup (150 g) blueberries
- 1 cup (150 g) red or yellow teardrop or cherry tomatoes (quarter the tomatoes if necessary, so they will be nearly the same size as the blueberries)
- ¼ cup (40 g) diced orange, red, or yellow bell pepper
- 1 tablespoon finely chopped fresh parsley
- 1 tablespoon chopped fresh cilantro
- 1 tablespoon honey
- 2 tablespoons avocado, pistachio, or walnut oil
- 2 tablespoons raspberry vinegar
- ½ tablespoon seeded and minced jalapeno or serrano chile
- Salt and pepper, to taste

1. Place the blueberries, tomatoes, and bell pepper in a large mixing bowl. No need to combine.

2. In a small bowl, whisk together the parsley, cilantro, honey, oil, vinegar, chile, salt, and pepper. Adjust the seasonings to your taste.

3. Pour the vinaigrette over the fruit and very gently combine the ingredients.

4. Allow the salsa to sit for twenty minutes before serving so flavors can blend.

5. Store in a covered container in the refrigerator for up to three days.

CRANBERRY SALSA WITH CILANTRO & CHILES

MAKES 3 CUPS (700 ML)

This is my favorite cranberry dish. Not only do I make it for the holidays, but also we often enjoy it during the fall and winter. It's a delicious way to get more cranberries into your diet and also gives you the health benefits of protein-and-zinc-rich pepitas and detoxifying onions and cilantro.

- ½ cup (70 g) pepitas (green shelled pumpkin seeds)
- 2 cups (200 g) fresh or frozen and thawed cranberries
- 1⅓ cups (135 g) chopped green onions (dark green parts only; about 2 bunches)
- 1 cup (50 g) chopped fresh cilantro

2 tablespoons minced seeded serrano chiles

6 tablespoons honey, coconut sugar, or regular sugar

6 tablespoons lime juice

1. Dry-toast the pepitas by placing them in a large skillet over high heat. After a minute you will hear popping and smell a delicious nutty smell. When that happens, turn off the heat and allow them to cool. Set aside.

2. Place the cranberries in a food processor and pulse until roughly chopped.

3. In a large bowl, gently combine onions, cilantro, and chiles, along with the chopped cranberries and dry-toasted pepitas.

4. In a small bowl, whisk together the honey and lime juice. Pour over the cranberry mixture and gently toss to mix.

5. Cover and chill for twenty minutes to allow flavors to blend.

6. Store in a covered container in the refrigerator for up to three days.

BERRY SALSA

MAKES 4 CUPS (1 L)

Berry salsa? It does sound kind of strange, doesn't it? But it's delicious—sweet, tart, savory, and refreshing—all at once. Oh, and the mix of antioxidant-rich berries and detoxifying cilantro are good for you too! This salsa is great with tortilla chips or on a quesadilla or cornmeal waffles, but it also pairs beautifully with grilled poultry, fish, and meats. It's best made right before serving.

1 cup (125 g) raspberries

1 cup (150 g) blueberries

1 cup (145 g) small blackberries or large blackberries cut in half

1 cup (190 g) strawberries, roughly chopped

¼ cup (40 g) red onion, chopped

¼ cup (5 g) chopped fresh cilantro

¼ cup (50 ml) honey

2 teaspoons lime juice

1. In a large bowl, combine the raspberries, blueberries, blackberries, strawberries, red onion, and cilantro. No need to combine at this point. Putting the ingredients in the bowl is enough.

2. In a small mixing bowl, whisk together the honey and lime juice.

3. Pour the honey-lime juice mixture over the fruit very, very gently so you don't break or puncture any of the berries, then gently toss all ingredients to combine.

4. Store in a covered container in the refrigerator for up to three days.

DIPS & SPREADS

BERRY HUMMUS

MAKES 4 CUPS (985 G)

Featuring berries, chickpeas, tahini, and orange juice, this high-protein, high-fiber recipe is unusual. It's also delicious. And fun. My kids like it slathered on tortillas or toast or as a dip for apples and carrot sticks. Give it a try!

- 3 cups (720 g) cooked chickpeas
- 4 tablespoons tahini
- 1 tablespoon walnut or extra-virgin olive oil
- 1½ cups (215 g) blackberries
- ¼ cup (50 ml) orange juice or unsweetened cranberry juice
- 2 tablespoons honey

1. Add the chickpeas, tahini, and oil to a food processor and process until smooth.

2. Add the berries, juice, and honey and pulse to blend.

3. Store in a covered container in the refrigerator for up to five days.

CRANBERRY–WHITE BEAN HUMMUS

MAKES 3½ CUPS (810 ML)

This unusual berry-based hummus includes cranberry sauce, making it a great treat for the holidays, when many of us have leftover cranberry sauce. Homemade sauce is awesome in this recipe, but you can use canned cranberry sauce—just make sure it's the whole berry variety and not the smooth gelatinous kind.

- 3 cups (530 g) cooked cannellini or great Northern beans, drained and rinsed
- Juice of 2 lemons
- ¼ cup (50 ml) walnut oil or extra-virgin olive oil
- 1 small garlic clove
- ¼ teaspoon ground cumin
- ¼ teaspoon salt
- ¼ teaspoon ground pepper
- 1½ teaspoons minced fresh sage
- ½ cup (140 g) whole berry cranberry sauce (Or you could use lingonberry sauce.)

1. In a food processor, combine beans, lemon juice, oil, garlic, cumin, salt, pepper, sage, and cranberry sauce until smooth.

2. Store in a covered container in the refrigerator for up to five days.

RED BERRY GUACAMOLE

MAKES ABOUT 2 CUPS (475 ML)

Guacamole! Isn't it great? It's healthy, too, thanks to glutathione-rich avocado, a food that contributes to brain and skin health. This tangy recipe features the sweet-tart charms of strawberry or raspberry (or you could even use red currants or lingonberries), which contribute a potent dose of vitamin C.

- *3 ripe medium Hass avocados*
- *Salt and pepper, to taste*
- *Juice of 1 lime or small lemon*
- *3 tablespoons chopped cilantro*
- *1 small jalapeno or habanero chile, seeded and minced*
- *1 small shallot, finely minced*
- *1 cup (145 g) ripe strawberries, roughly chopped, or raspberries*

1. Scoop the avocado into a large bowl and add the salt and pepper, lime juice, cilantro, jalapeno, and shallot. Using a potato masher or the back of a large fork, mash the ingredients until somewhat smooth.

2. Fold in the berries and adjust the seasoning.

3. Serve immediately.

AVOCADOS: THE SEXY SUPERFOOD

Delicious, yes, but also nutritious! Avocados are bursting with a wide range of health-boosting benefits.

- One cup of avocado has over 35 percent of one's daily allowance for vitamin K, a vitamin associated with bone formation and proper blood clotting, as well as the transport of calcium through the body.

- Avocados help the body absorb other nutrients. For instance, one cup of fresh avocado, when eaten with another food, can increase the body's absorption of carotenoids from that food between 200 and 400 percent.

- One cup of avocado supplies 30 percent of the daily recommendation of fiber.

- Avocados are a powerful anti-inflammatory food, boasting a range of phytoerols, carotenoids, antioxidants, and omega-3 fatty acids, all of which help prevent or lessen arthritis, cardiovascular disease, and autoimmune diseases.

- Avocado has been found to help prevent the occurrence of cancers of the mouth, skin, and prostate gland, probably due to its antioxidant-boosting ability and high content of anti-inflammatory nutrients.

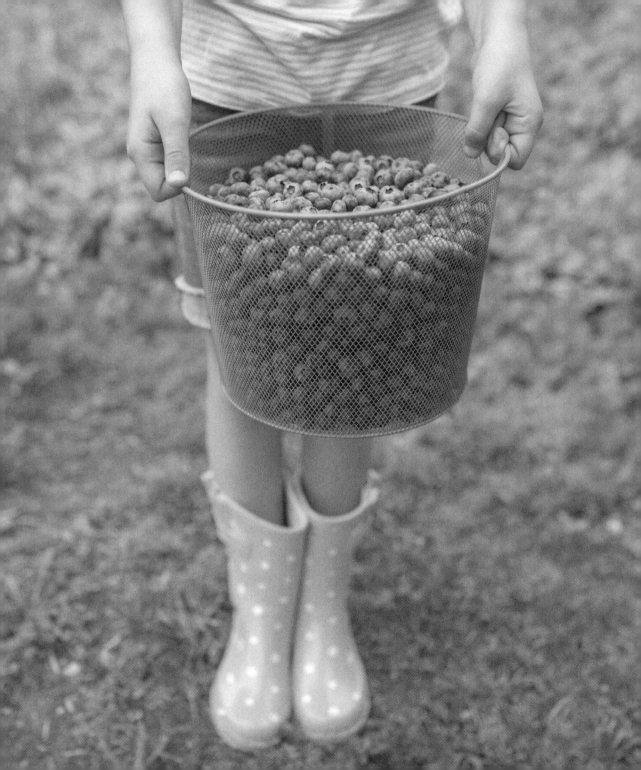

CHAPTER 10

FREQUENTLY ASKED QUESTIONS

Humans have been eating berries of all kinds since the beginning of time. That doesn't mean we know everything about them, though. Here are some of the most common questions about berries.

What makes something a berry?

From a culinary standpoint, a berry is a small, juicy fruit. But the botanical definition is decidedly narrower: In scientific terms, a berry is a fruit produced from the ovary of a single flower in which the outer layer of the ovary wall develops into a pericarp (a fleshy portion). If you choose to go by the botanical definition, you can count tomatoes, cucumbers, and bananas as berries.

What country grows the most strawberries?

China. According to the most recent statistics available from the Food and Agriculture Organization of the United Nations (2013), China produced the most strawberries (2,997,504 metric tons), followed by the United States (1,360,869 metric tons), Mexico (379,464 metric tons), Turkey (372,498 metric tons), and Spain (312,500 metric tons).

How about raspberries?

The Russian Federation (133,000 metric tons), followed by Poland (127,055 metric tons), the United States (100,755 metric tons), Serbia (96,078 metric tons), Ukraine (30,300 metric tons), and Mexico (17,009 metric tons).

And blueberries?

In 2012, the United States produced 255,827 metric tons of blueberries, Chile produced about 94,801 metric tons, and Canada produced about 48,081 metric tons.

How do I know if a wild berry is poisonous?

There isn't a reliable way to know if an unfamiliar berry is poisonous. Your best defense against poisonous berries is to avoid putting unknown fruit in your mouth!

Why can birds and other animals eat berries that are poisonous to humans?

It's believed that deer, bears, birds, and other wild animals can eat plants that contain neurotoxins because they have slightly different nerve receptors than humans do. Also, animals have different symbiotic bacteria in their digestive tract than humans, which helps them break down and digest the vegetation they eat.

I grow my own berries. Is there a way I can keep birds and other animals from eating them?

A lot of creatures—humans included—love berries, which is why a bramble of blackberries or raspberries, a strawberry patch, or a thicket of any type of berry, for that matter, attracts all types of animals. The good news is you can use a few measures to ensure that your berries aren't devoured before you have a chance to pick them. The bad news is that none of these methods is 100 percent foolproof:

- Use netting over the plants to minimize the number of berries deer and birds eat. Be aware, though, that some small birds and animals can get beneath it.

- Plant twice as many berry bushes as you think you'll need, thus ensuring you'll have enough berries for your needs.

- Tie strips of metallic material, called Reflective Bird Scare Tape (available in garden centers), to bushes and plants to scare away birds and other animals.

- Make your own "scare product" by tying CDs and/or aluminum pie plates to branches.

- Post a few faux owls (available at garden centers) among the plants.

- Hang several bird feeders near your berries, giving the birds something else to enjoy. Just make sure to keep the feeders full. Birds will return again and again to them. If the feeders are empty, your winged friends will make a beeline for your berries.

Can eating too many berries be harmful to my health?

Probably not, although eating more than a cup of berries in a sitting does cause diarrhea (with strong cramping) in some individuals. Berries are a particularly good choice for those with diabetes, who may worry about fruit: Berries are lower in fructose than bananas, melons, mangoes, and other fruits. Studies also suggest that a serving of raspberries, blackberries, red currants, or strawberries each day can reduce diabetic symptoms. (These studies are mentioned in Chapter 2.) Before increasing your berry consumption, however, be safe and speak with your health-care provider.

Are frozen berries as healthy as fresh berries?

Yes. And in some cases, frozen berries are more nutrient dense than the fresh berries you find in the produce section of your local market. Why? It has to do with time. The longer a berry sits around (maybe on a truck traveling from a farm to your local market), the more nutrients it loses. Frozen fruit is usually frozen on site, only moments after it's been picked, literally locking in nutrients. This has been proven by several studies, including a July 2014 study from the University of South Dakota published in *Science Daily*, that found that a group of antioxidant compounds in blueberries and other berries, called anthocyanins, become more bioavailable when frozen. This is a great reason to keep a few bags of berries in your freezer.

Why are berries considered superfood? Is it because they have fiber, vitamins, and minerals?

The fiber, vitamins, and minerals in berries (of all kinds) make them a very healthy food. However, what makes them a superfood are phytonutrients, powerful antioxidants helping to strengthen the immune system, heal and prevent heart conditions, create a strong nervous system, protect against cancer, heal the skin and eyes, and so much more.

Can you talk a bit more about phytonutrients?

Plant foods contain vitamins and minerals that are essential to keeping humans alive. Plants also contain something that—while not essential to human life—helps prevent disease and keep our bodies working properly. These are plant chemicals called phytonutrients, or phytochemicals. They help protect plants from bacteria, viruses, germs, fungi, bugs, drought, and temperature fluctuations. It is believed that more than 25,000 phytonutrients are found in plant foods. Six of the most important phytonutrients include carotenoids, ellagic acid, flavonoids, resveratrol, glucosinolates, and phytoestrogens.

I know that many popular berries are actually crosses between two types of berries. How do scientists do this?

Sometimes it is Mother Nature's doing. For instance, a California farmer planted raspberries near wild blackberries and a new plant sprung up, which he named Loganberry (after himself). Boysenberries were born when Loganberries were grown near a wild berry called the Easter dewberry. Scientists can artificially create new varieties by choosing a male plant of another variety and artificially "inseminating" a female plant of another variety.

BERRY ASSOCIATIONS

www.njcranberries.org
Based in New Jersey, this is the official site of the American Cranberry Growers Association.

www.blueberries.com/
The Blueberry People® MBG Marketing offers a wealth of information on this berry.

www.bcgojigrowersassociation.webnode.com/
BC Goji Growers Association is a Canadian-based organization that helps North American goji growers.

www.crfg.org/
California Rare Fruit Growers, Inc., is a great place to find information on berries (such as red and black currants and elderberries) that are not commonly grown commercially.

www.cranberryinstitute.org/
The Cranberry Institute is dedicated to supporting research on the health benefits of cranberries.

www.elderberrygrowers.org/
This is the page for the Midwest Elderberry Association. Membership is open to those interested in elderberry culture.

www.nationalberrycrops.org/
The National Berry Crops Initiative is a partnership of industry, academia, and government organizations.

www.nasga.org/
The North American Strawberry Growers Association represents more than 250 members in forty states, ten Canadian provinces, and fifteen countries.

www.ontarioberries.com/
The Ontario Berry Growers Association features commercially popular berries, as well as less-grown fruits, such as gooseberries and currants.

www.raspberryblackberry.com/
At the official site of the North American Raspberry & Blackberry Association, you will find a consumer-information page about these berries from finding farms to health and nutrition benefits.

www.unitedcranberry.com/
Visit this site to learn more about the United Cranberry Growers Cooperative.

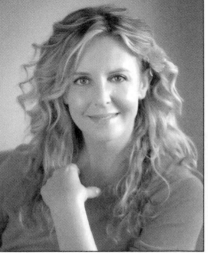

PHOTO BY ALYSSA POLCEK-PEEK

STEPHANIE PEDERSEN is a holistic nutritionist, food educator, cookbook author, corporate speaker, and media host. The author of more than twenty-two books, Stephanie has a reputation for teaching people how to make nutrition easy, practical, and fun. She does this by using superfoods and other "power foods" to help individuals detoxify naturally, manage food allergies, eliminate cravings, and lose weight using food and lifestyle changes.

Pedersen currently lives in New York City with her husband and three sons. Visit her at www.StephaniePedersen.com for free gifts and classes, as well as to learn more about using foods and lifestyle actions to make your life healthier and happier. You can also learn more by tuning in to one of Stephanie's weekly radio shows—*Your Big Life* and *The Superfood Moment*—or stop by YouTube for her family health series, *Real Eating*, starring Stephanie and her sons.

ALSO BY STEPHANIE PEDERSEN:

The 7-Day Superfood Cleanse

Coconut: The Complete Guide to the World's Most Versatile Superfood

Kale: The Complete Guide to the World's Most Powerful Superfood

The Pumpkin Pie Spice Cookbook

KISS Guide to Beauty: Keep It Simple Series

Garlic: Safe and Effective Self-Care for Arthritis, High Blood Pressure, and Flu

ACKNOWLEDGMENTS

I couldn't have finished *Berries: The Complete Guide to Cooking with Power-Packed Berries* without the support of many special people. First, a shout-out to my sons, Leif Christian Pedersen, Anders Gyldenvalde Pedersen, and Axel SuneLund Pedersen. Your mother is crazy. Yes, I know that you know that, but I want you to remember that writing a book does strange things to a person! Thank you for your patience, for your humor, and for being the thoughtful young men that you are.

Continuing that train of thought: hubby Richard Demler, wow, what a year, huh? It's been great seeing you dive in to life and grow bigger and more powerful.

Thanks to so many friends who supported my family and me during the book-writing process. Oceana, you are my favorite goddess. Our morning check-ins are so powerful. Lola, through thick and thin, you continue to be a rock; I am so grateful for you.

I want to give a shout-out to the Saint Thomas Choir School for taking such outstanding care of Leif and Anders as I wrote—headmaster, housemothers, choir directors, organists, teachers, gap students, school chef, and all of you. Your just-watchful-enough eyes and encouragement perfectly supported my kids, freeing up the mental energy I needed to write. And thanks too to my choir-school parent friends who have become family: You rock. Kathleen Rhodes, I just want to say thank you. Your sense of adventure is thrilling, your fierce dedication to our boys' education inspires me, and your steadfastness amazes me. You have played a role in my kids' success, all while juggling seemingly insurmountable challenges in your own world. Plus, you are the best road-trip partner ever! Godmother Dina Erickson, your exquisite care and championing of Leif and Anders and Axel have made you their favorite mother of all

time. I appreciate you and your hilarious hubby, my kids' godfather, Peter Erickson.

Thanks to my amazing clients for the constant inspiration you bring. I am in awe of each of you!

I can't say enough flattering (and true!) things about editor Jennifer Williams. We go back in time through several publishing houses now. I count my blessings that I was assigned, as a young author, to you all of those years ago. Here's to us!

I am grateful for my designer, Barbara Balch, who ensured that this book is as polished and professional looking as it is! Bill Milne created the gorgeous, mouthwatering photos in *Berries: The Complete Guide to Cooking with Power-Packed Berries.* And my very thorough production editor, Kimberly Broderick, kept us all on schedule, while seeing to all the details with her usual equanimity and patience. Thank you! Your calm can-do demeanor and overall smarty-pants ways make this crazy business of publishing look glamorous.

Thanks so much to my publicity pro, Sherri McClendon, of Professional Moneta. Sherri, I adore our monthly conversations. Not only are you fun and witty (and you know how much I love witty people), you make my professional life so much easier!

Lastly, I must thank you, dear reader, for your love of berries! Thank you!

INDEX

Note: When looking up recipes by berry type, see also "Berries (various), recipes with."

A

Acai, 8–12
  about: general information, 11–12, 64; health-supporting role, 10–11, 64; nutrition profile, 8–10; storing, 11; things to be aware of, 12; using/uses, 11, 12, 64
Acai Berry Breakfast Bowl, 86
Creamy Acai Dressing, 100
Alcohol. See Cocktails and mocktails
Amino acids, 9
Antioxidant power, 4, 14, 18, 19, 38, 66. See also Free radicals; Phytonutrients; Vitamin A; Vitamin C; Vitamin E
Apples
  about: making apple sauce, 131
  Blueberry-Cabbage Power Juice, 59
  Granola Cookies, 81
  Morning Glory Juice, 60
  Winter Berry Juice, 60
Avocados
  about: nutritional benefits, 173
  Alpha Omega Salad, 94–95
  Avocado-Bean-Berry Sandwich, 104
  Berry-Avocado Ice Cream, 158
  Berry Avocado Pudding, 145
  Key Lime-Avocado Berry Pie, 153
  Mango Goji Avocado Salsa, 169
  Red Berry Guacamole, 173

B

Baked Berry Oatmeal, 84
Barley, curried cranberry, 136–137
Bars and bites. See Snacks
Beans and other legumes
  Autumn Salad, 96–97
  Avocado-Bean-Berry Sandwich, 104
  Berry Hummus, 172
  Berry Main-Dish Salad Blueprint, 119–120
  Black Bean Blueberry Bowl, 101
  Cranberry-White Bean Hummus, 172
  Raspberry Buffalo Slow Cooker Chili, 89–90
  Slow Cooker Berry-Bean Sloppy Joes, 118, 124
Bearberries, 14
Beef and bison
  Berry Main-Dish Salad Blueprint, 119–120
  Blueberry Sliders, 127
  Raspberry Buffalo Slow Cooker Chili, 89–90
  Red Currant Cocoa Stew, 91
Berries

benefits, iv
consumption statistics, v–vi, 4, 103
cross-pollinated, 177
definition of, 1, 175
frozen, healthiness of, 177
general appeal of, vii
historical perspective, 1–3, 4
increasing appeal of, v–vi, 3–4
measurements/conversions, 73
poisonous, 175–176
questions and answers, 175–177
storing. See Storing berries
superfood status, 177
this book and, 4
Berries (various), recipes with
  about: low-sugar jams recipe, 85
  Acai Berry Breakfast Bowl, 86
  Baked Berry Oatmeal, 84
  Balsamic Berries, 143
  Banana Berry Omelet, 87
  Berry-Avocado Ice Cream, 158
  Berry Breakfast Polenta, 82
  Berry Coconut Age-Fighting Mask, 127
  Berry Granita, 158
  Berry Iced Tea, 67
  Berry Main-Dish Salad Blueprint, 119–120
  Berry Red Quinoa Pilaf, 135
  Berry Salad Dressing Blueprint, 120
  Berry Salsa, 171
  Berry Side-Dish Salad Blueprint, 120
  Berry Sorbet, 157
  Bright & Bubbly, 68
  Coconut Berry Pops, 116
  Coconut Water Berry Pops, 117
  Ginger Berry Switchel, 56
  Homemade Berry Syrup, 58
  Mixed Berry Coulis, 159
  Smooth Berry Soup, 144
  White Berry Tea, 61
  Whole Berry Gelatin, 106, 114–115
Biotin, 49
Bison, in Raspberry Buffalo Slow Cooker Chili, 89–90
Black currants. See Currants, black
Blackberries, 12–16
  about: buying, 15; general information, 15–16, 83; health-supporting role, 14–15, 16, 66, 83; nutrition profile, 12–14; storing, 15–16; things to be aware of, 16; using/uses, 16
  Berry Breakfast Syrup, 78
  Berry Crème Parfait, 144
  Berry Hummus, 172
  Berry Melon Sparkler, 72
  Berry Nut Butter Pocket, 103
  Berry Sangria, 71
  Berry Slump, 154

Black Rice Bowl, 100–101
Blackberry-Cabbage Power Juice, 59
Blackberry Cucumber Water, 55
Blackberry Green Beans, 137–138
Blackberry Mint Iced Tea, 66
Blackberry Mustard, 164
Blackberry Scrub for Face & Body, 122
Chicken with Berry Sauce, 129–130
Chocolate-Berry Pots de Crème, 146
Chocolate-Berry Torte, 151
Multi-Berry Luncheon Salad, 96
Pulled Pork Surprise Wrap, 105
Superfood Purple Smoothie, 57
Blood pressure, lowering, 22, 38. See also Potassium; Vitamin C
Blood sugar, lowering, 11, 17, 39–40, 41, 42, 49–50. See also Fiber; Manganese
Blood vessels, healing, 39
Blueberries, 16–19
  about: buying, 18; consumption statistics, v–vi; general information, 18–19, 99, 175; health-supporting role, 17–18, 70; nutrition profile, 17; storing, 18; things to be aware of, 19; using/uses, 18, 19
  Alpha Omega Salad, 94–95
  Baked Berry Oatmeal, 84
  Berry Bombs, 109–110
  Berry Breakfast Quinoa, 83
  Berry Kale Quinoa, 135
  Berry Nut Butter Pocket, 103
  Berry Omelet, 87
  Berry Pork Chops, 128
  Berry Sangria, 71
  Black Bean Blueberry Bowl, 101
  Blueberry Banana Oatmeal Bread, 75–76
  Blueberry Barbecue Sauce, 166–167
  Blueberry Bellini, 70
  Blueberry Breakfast Cookies, 148
  Blueberry-Cabbage Power Juice, 59
  Blueberry Chicken Salad Sandwich, 104–105
  Blueberry Chocolate Clusters, 160–161
  Blueberry Chutney, 167
  Blueberry Crisp, 155
  Blueberry Fluff, 145
  Blueberry Sliders, 127
  Blueberry Tart, 142, 152
  Blueberry Turmeric Acne Mask, 149
  Coconut Water Berry Pops, 117
  Easy Curry-Berry Ketchup, 164
  Flourless PB&B Cookies, 148–149

Fruity Salmon, 131
Gluten-Free Blueberry Corn Muffins, 76
Granola Cookies, 81
Herbal Berry Millet, 136
Homemade Vegan Blueberry Granola Bars, 110–111
Multi-Berry Luncheon Salad, 96
No-Bake Blueberry-Coconut Bars, 107
Spicy Berry Greens, 140
Spicy Berry Ketchup, 165
Superfood Purple Smoothie, 57
Turkey Tenderloin with Cranberry-Shallot Sauce, 128–129
Bowls, 86, 100–101
Brain function, improving, 15, 36, 70. See also Omega-3 fatty acids
Brain function, Parkinson's disease and, 42, 45–46, 94, 158, 173
Breads and cakes, morning
  Berry Breakfast Syrup for, 78
  Blueberry Banana Oatmeal Bread, 75–76
  Gluten-Free Blueberry Corn Muffins, 76
  Gluten-Free Coconut-Berry Waffles, 74, 77–78
  Paleo-Style Strawberry Pancakes, 77
Breakfast, 75–87. See also Breads and cakes, morning
  Acai Berry Breakfast Bowl, 86
  Baked Berry Oatmeal, 84
  Banana Berry Omelet, 87
  Berry Breakfast Polenta, 82
  Berry Breakfast Quinoa, 83
  Berry Breakfast Syrup, 78
  Berry Omelet, 87
  Blueberry Breakfast Cookies, 148
  Granola Cookies, 81
  Nut-Free High Protein Granola, 80
  Nuts & Seeds Granola, 79
  Strawberry Chia Pudding, 86
Brussels sprouts, 141

C

Cabbage, in juice, 59
Calcium, 9, 13
Cancer
  fighting/killing cells, 10, 15, 24, 39, 43
  free radicals and, 18. See also Free radicals
  preventing/reducing risk, 8, 12, 14, 15, 26, 27, 28, 36–37, 50, 59, 68, 169, 173. See also Fiber
  reducing tumors, 42
  vitamin C and, 49
Candy, 160–161
Celery, in Raspberry Celery Smoothie, 57
Cereal. See Breakfast

Chicken. *See* Poultry
Chili, raspberry buffalo, 89–90
Chocolate
    Blueberry Chocolate Clusters,
        160–161
    Chocolate-Berry Pots de Crème,
        146
    Chocolate-Berry Torte, 151
    Chocolate-Dipped Strawberries,
        160
    Dark Chocolate Superfood
        Bark, 161
    Red Currant Cocoa Stew, 91
Chokeberries, 19
Cholesterol, 9, 11, 14, 18, 41–42, 50,
    63, 93, 108, 169
Choline, 14
Cilantro, benefits of, 93
Citrus
    Berry Herbal Tea with Orange
        Spices, 65
    Fruity Chia Pops, 115
    Key Lime-Avocado Berry Pie,
        153
    Morning Glory Juice, 60
    Sparkling Raspberry Limeade, 69
Cloud berries, 19
Cocktails and mocktails, 68–73
    about: berry ice cubes, 56;
        mocktails, 68–69; muddling,
        55
    Berry Melon Sparkler, 72
    Berry Sangria, 71
    Blueberry Bellini, 70
    Bright & Bubbly, 68
    Cranberry Fizz, 69
    Scandinavian Spritzer, 71
    Sparkling Raspberry Limeade, 69
    Strawberry-Rosé Spritzer, 72
    Watermelon Strawberry Sipper,
        68
Coconut
    about: milk of, 146
    Berry Bombs, 109–110
    Berry Coconut Age-Fighting
        Mask, 127
    Coconut Berry Pops, 116
    Coconut Water Berry Pops, 117
    Gluten-Free Coconut-Berry
        Waffles, 74, 77–78
    No-Bake Blueberry-Coconut
        Bars, 107
    Quinoa Coconut Chicken Bowl,
        88, 102
    Whipped Coconut Cream, 150
Condiments. *See* Sauces and
    condiments; Syrups
Copper, 9, 14, 17, 21, 44, 49, 79, 108
Corn muffins, gluten-free blueberry,
    76
Cough syrup, 62–63
Cranberries, 19–24
    about: buying, 22–23; general
        information, 22–24, 103;
        health-supporting role,
        21–22, 69; juice warning,
        61; nutrition profile, 19–21;

storing, 23; things to be aware
    of, 24, 61; using/uses, 23, 24
Acorn Squash with Walnuts &
    Cranberries, 126
Almond-Berry Shortbread, 147
Baked Berry Oatmeal, 84
Berry Bombs, 109–110
Berry Herbal Tea with Orange
    Spices, 65
Berry Red Quinoa Pilaf, 135
Brussels Sprouts with Walnuts
    and Dried Cranberries, 141
Cranberry Drink, 62
Cranberry Fizz, 69
Cranberry Relish, 168
Cranberry Salsa with Cilantro
    and Chiles, 170–171
Cranberry-White Bean Hummus,
    172
Curried Cranberry Barley,
    136–137
Dark Chocolate Superfood
    Bark, 161
DIY Cranberry Raw Food Bars,
    108
Flourless PB&B Cookies,
    148–149
Granola Cookies, 81
Mashed Sweet Potatoes with
    Berries, 138–139
Mulled Berry Tea, 64
Nut-Free High Protein Granola,
    80
Nuts & Seeds Granola, 79
Quinoa Cranberry Red Soup, 92
Sparkling Berry Cooler, 53
Spicy Berry Greens, 140
Tangy Cranberry Dressing, 98
Turkey Tenderloin with
    Cranberry-Shallot Sauce,
    128–129
Winter Berry Juice, 60
Cucumbers
    Blackberry Cucumber Water, 55
    Blueberry-Cabbage Power
        Juice, 59
    Cucumber and Gooseberry Soup,
        93–94
    Morning Glory Juice, 60
Cumin, nutritional benefits, 90
Currants, black
    about, 24–27; buying, 26; general
        information, 26–27, 126;
        health-supporting role,
        25–26; nutrition profile,
        24–25, 126; storing, 26;
        using/uses, 26, 27
    Black Currant Sauce, 132–133
    Chocolate-Berry Pots de Crème,
        146
    Sweet & Sour Black Currant
        Sauce, 163–164
Currants, red, 27–29
    about: buying, 29; general
        information, 29, 131; health-
        supporting role, 28; nutrition
        profile, 27–28; storing, 29;

things to be aware of, 29;
    using/uses, 29
All Things Red Gazpacho, 121
Red Currant & Rosemary
    Chutney, 168
Red Currant Cocoa Stew, 91
Red Currant Sauce, 134

D
Dates, nutritional benefits, 108
Desserts, 143–159. *See also*
    Chocolate; Snacks
    Almond-Berry Shortbread, 147
    Balsamic Berries, 143
    Berry-Avocado Ice Cream, 158
    Berry Avocado Pudding, 145
    Berry Crème Parfait, 144
    Berry Granita, 158
    Berry Shortcake Biscuits, 149–150
    Berry Slump, 154
    Berry Sorbet, 157
    Blueberry Breakfast Cookies, 148
    Blueberry Crisp, 155
    Blueberry Fluff, 145
    Blueberry Tart, 142, 152
    Flourless PB&B Cookies, 148–149
    Key Lime-Avocado Berry Pie,
        153
    Mixed Berry Coulis, 159
    Red Cobbler, 156
    Smooth Berry Soup, 144
    Whipped Coconut Cream, 150
Diabetes, 28, 30, 36, 176. *See also*
    Blood sugar, lowering; Insulin
    resistance
Dinner, 119–141. *See also* Grain
    sides; Vegetarian main dishes;
    Veggie sides
    about: berry dinner sauces,
        132–134; overview of recipes,
        119
    All Things Red Gazpacho, 121
    Berry Main-Dish Salad
        Blueprint, 119–120
    Berry Pork Chops, 128
    Berry Salad Dressing Blueprint,
        120
    Berry Side-Dish Salad Blueprint,
        120
    Blueberry Sliders, 127
    Chicken with Berry Sauce,
        129–130
    Curried Halibut with Raspberry-
        Mango Relish, 130
    Fruity Salmon, 131
    Goji Berry Soup, 122
    Spicy Strawberry Gazpacho, 121
    Turkey Tenderloin with
        Cranberry-Shallot Sauce,
        128–129
Dips and spreads, 172–173
Drinks, 53–69. *See also* Cocktails and
    mocktails; Teas
    about: cranberry juice warning,
        61; muddling, 55; sparkly
        water types (carbonated,
        seltzer, mineral, etc.), 54

Blackberry Cucumber Water, 55
Blueberry-Cabbage Power
    Juice, 59
Ginger Berry Switchel, 56
Morning Glory Juice, 60
Raspberry Celery Smoothie, 57
Sparkling Berry Cooler, 53
Strawberry Basil Soda, 55
Superfood Purple Smoothie, 57
Winter Berry Juice, 60

E
Edamame Strawberry Stew, 125
Egg omelets, 87
Elderberries, 29–32
    about: buying, 31; general
        information, 31–32, 140;
        health-supporting role, 30–
        31; nutrition profile, 29–30;
        storing, 32; things to be aware
        of, 32; using/uses, 32
    Elderberry Sauce, 132
    Elderberry Syrup, 62–63
Exercise, recovery after, 25
Eyesight, improving, 17–18, 46, 134,
    139. *See also* Glaucoma

F
Facial care. *See* Skin care
Fiber, 8, 12, 13, 17, 20, 27, 30, 33, 35,
    38, 41, 44, 48
Fish and seafood
    Alpha Omega Salad, 94–95
    Berry Main-Dish Salad
        Blueprint, 119–120
    Curried Halibut with Raspberry-
        Mango Relish, 130
    Fruity Salmon, 131
Flu, warding off, 30–31, 62–63
Folate (vitamin B9), 13, 14, 44, 49
Free radicals, 10, 18, 20, 30, 36, 40,
    41, 44, 66
Frozen snacks. *See* Snacks
Fungal infections, treating, 31

G
Gazpachos, 121
Gelatin, whole berry and variations,
    106, 114–115
Ginger Berry Switchel, 56
Glaucoma, 25–26
Gluten-Free Blueberry Corn
    Muffins, 76
Gluten-Free Coconut-Berry Waffles,
    74, 77–78
Goji berries, 32–35
    about: buying, 34; general
        information, 34–35; health-
        supporting role, 33–34, 80;
        hydrated berry uses, 65;
        nutrition profile, 32–33;
        storing, 34; things to be aware
        of, 35; using/uses, 34–35, 65
    Autumn Salad, 96–97
    Berry Bombs, 109–110
    Dark Chocolate Superfood
        Bark, 161
    Flourless PB&B Cookies,
        148–149

Goji Berry Soup, 122
Goji Berry Tea, 65
Goji Spaghetti Squash, 139
Goji Strawberry Vinaigrette
    Dressing, 98
Mango Goji Avocado Salsa, 169
Nut-Free High Protein Granola,
    80
Nut-Free Protein Bites, 109
Nuts & Seeds Granola, 79
Slow Cooker Berry-Bean Sloppy
    Joes, 118, 124
Smothered Sweet Potatoes, 123
Spicy Berry Greens, 140
Super Berry Fruit Leather,
    112–113
Superfood Salad, 95
Turkey Tenderloin with
    Cranberry-Shallot Sauce,
    128–129
Golden berries, 36
Golden Berry Salad Dressing, 99
Gooseberries, 35–38
    about: buying, 37; general
        information, 37–38, 94;
        health-supporting role, 36–
        37; nutrition profile, 35–37;
        storing, 37; things to be aware
        of, 38; using/uses, 37, 38
    Cucumber and Gooseberry Soup,
        93–94
    Gooseberry Papaya Face Pack,
        141
    Gooseberry Sauce, 134
Grain sides, 135–137
    Berry Kale Quinoa, 135
    Berry Red Quinoa Pilaf, 135
    Curried Cranberry Barley,
        136–137
    Herbal Berry Millet, 136
Grains, breakfast. See Breakfast
Granola. See Oats
Green beans, blackberry, 137–138
Greens, spicy berry, 140
Growing berries, 176. See also specific
    berries, general information
Gut health. See also Fiber;
    Inflammation, reducing

H
Hawthorn berries, 38
Hawthorn Berry Tea, 63
Health benefits, overview of, vi–
    vii, 7. See also Therapeutic
    recipes; specific berries; specific
    conditions
Heart health, 28, 46. See also
    Hawthorn berries; Omega-3
    fatty acids; Potassium
Hemorrhoids, 33, 83
History of berries, 1–3, 4. See
    also specific berries, general
    information
Huckleberries, 39

I
Ice cubes, berry, 56
Immune system, strengthening/

improving, 10, 19, 33–34.
    See also Fiber; Manganese;
    Vitamin A; Vitamin B6;
    Vitamin C; Vitamin E
Inflammation, reducing, 36, 37,
    39, 46, 50, 63, 93, 108, 126,
    173. See also Phytonutrients;
    Selenium
IBD, 22
    intestinal, 21. See also Fiber
    vascular, 26
Influenza, warding off, 30–31, 62–63
Insulin resistance, 21. See also
    Diabetes
Iodine, 49
Iron, 9, 13, 25, 30, 33, 41, 79, 90

J
Juices, 59–61

K
Kale, 95, 135
Ketchups, 164–165

L
Leather, fruit, 111–113
Lingonberries, 38–41
    about: buying, 40; general
        information, 40–41; health-
        supporting role, 39–40;
        nutrition profile, 38–39;
        storing, 40; things to be aware
        of, 40; using/uses, 40, 41
    All Things Red Gazpacho, 121
    Lingonberry Sauce, 133
    Scandinavian Spritzer, 71
Lunch, 89–105. See also Salads;
    Soups and stews; Wraps and
    sandwiches
    about: berries at, 89
    Black Bean Blueberry Bowl, 101
    Black Rice Bowl, 100–101
    Quinoa Coconut Chicken Bowl,
        88, 102

M
Magnesium, 9, 13, 45, 47, 49, 79, 108
Manganese, 9, 14, 17, 21, 25, 28, 36,
    44–45, 49, 108, 111
Mango
    about: nutritional benefits, 169
    Fruity Chia Pops, 115
    Mango Goji Avocado Salsa, 169
    Quinoa Coconut Chicken Bowl,
        88, 102
    Raspberry Celery Smoothie, 57
    Raspberry-Mango Relish, 130
Masks. See Skin care
Measuring berry quantities, 73
Melon, 68, 72
Memory, blueberry juice for, 70
Millet, herbal berry, 136
Minerals, generous source of, 11. See
    also specific minerals
Mint blackberry iced tea, 66
Mocktails, 68–69
Mulberries, 41–43
    about: buying, 42; general
        information, 42–43, 113;
        health-supporting role,

41–42; nutrition profile, 41;
        storing, 42–43; things to be
        aware of, 43; using/uses, 43
    Mulberry Face Pack, 156
    Mulberry Salad Dressing, 97
    Super Berry Fruit Leather,
        112–113

N
Niacin, 13
Nutrition profiles. See specific berries;
    specific nutrients
Nuts and seeds
    Acai Berry Breakfast Bowl, 86
    Acorn Squash with Walnuts &
        Cranberries, 126
    Almond-Berry Shortbread, 147
    Alpha Omega Salad, 94–95
    Baked Berry Oatmeal, 84
    Berry Bombs, 109–110
    Berry Kale Quinoa, 135
    Berry Nut Butter Pocket, 103
    Black Rice Bowl, 100–101
    Blueberry Banana Oatmeal
        Bread, 75–76
    Blueberry Chicken Salad
        Sandwich, 104–105
    Blueberry Fluff, 145
    Brussels Sprouts with Walnuts
        and Dried Cranberries, 141
    Creamy Acai Dressing, 100
    Dark Chocolate Superfood
        Bark, 161
    DIY Cranberry Raw Food
        Bars, 108
    Flourless PB&B Cookies,
        148–149
    Fruity Chia Pops, 115
    Fruity Nut Butter Pops, 117
    Gluten-Free Coconut-Berry
        Waffles, 74, 77–78
    Granola Cookies, 81
    Homemade Vegan Blueberry
        Granola Bars, 110–111
    Multi-Berry Luncheon Salad, 96
    Nut-Free Protein Bites, 109
    Nuts & Seeds Granola, 79
    Quinoa Coconut Chicken Bowl,
        88, 102
    Spicy Berry Greens, 140
    Strawberry and Almond Fruit
        Roll-Ups, 113–114
    Strawberry Chia Pudding, 86
    Super Berry Fruit Leather,
        112–113
    Superfood Salad, 95

O
Oats
    about: nutritional benefits, 79
    Baked Berry Oatmeal, 84
    Berry Bombs, 109–110
    Blueberry Banana Oatmeal
        Bread, 75–76
    Blueberry Breakfast Cookies, 148
    Granola Cookies, 81
    Homemade Vegan Blueberry
        Granola Bars, 110–111

Nut-Free High Protein Granola,
    80
Nuts & Seeds Granola, 79
Obesity, fighting, 21
Omega-3 fatty acids, 8, 24, 27, 30,
    44, 48, 94, 131
Oral health, 15
Oxidative stress, 28, 34, 40

P
Pancakes, strawberry, 77
Pantothenic acid (vitamin B5), 21, 45
Papaya, in Gooseberry Papaya Face
    Pack, 141
Parkinson's disease, supporting, 42
Pear sauce, 131
Phosphorus, 9, 13, 49, 79
Phytonutrients, 17, 21, 23, 25, 28, 29,
    31, 36, 37, 39, 177
Polenta, berry breakfast, 82
Pops. See Snacks
Pork dishes, 105, 119–120, 128
Potassium, 9, 13, 25, 28, 30, 41, 45,
    47, 49, 108
Poultry
    Berry Main-Dish Salad
        Blueprint, 119–120
    Blueberry Chicken Salad
        Sandwich, 104–105
    Chicken with Berry Sauce,
        129–130
    Goji Berry Soup, 122
    Pulled Chicken (Pork) Surprise
        Wrap, 105
    Quinoa Coconut Chicken Bowl,
        88, 102
    Turkey Tenderloin with
        Cranberry-Shallot Sauce,
        128–129
Protein, 8, 12, 13, 24, 27, 29–30, 32,
    35, 38, 80. See also Amino
    acids
Protein bites, nut-free, 109

Q
Quinoa
    Berry Bombs, 109–110
    Berry Breakfast Quinoa, 83
    Berry Kale Quinoa, 135
    Berry Red Quinoa Pilaf, 135
    Nut-Free Protein Bites, 109
    Quinoa Coconut Chicken Bowl,
        88, 102
    Quinoa Cranberry Red Soup, 92
    Superfood Salad, 95

R
Raspberries, 44–48
    about: blue raspberry origins,
        115; buying, 46; general
        information, 46–48, 115,
        175; health-supporting role,
        45–46; nutrition profile,
        44–45; storing, 46–47; things
        to be aware of, 47; using/
        uses, 47, 48
    All Things Red Gazpacho, 121
    Berry Avocado Pudding, 145
        (continued)

(continued from previous page)
Berry Crème Parfait, 144
Berry Nut Butter Pocket, 103
Berry Sangria, 71
Chocolate-Berry Pots de Crème, 146
Chocolate-Berry Torte, 151
Coconut Water Berry Pops, 117
Fruity Chia Pops, 115
Fruity Salmon, 131
Herbal Berry Millet, 136
Key Lime-Avocado Berry Pie, 153
Mulled Berry Tea, 64
Multi-Berry Luncheon Salad, 96
Quinoa Coconut Chicken Bowl, 88, 102
Raspberry Buffalo Slow Cooker Chili, 89–90
Raspberry Celery Smoothie, 57
Raspberry-Mango Relish, 130
Raspberry Wrinkle Softener, 155
Red Berry Guacamole, 173
Red Cobbler, 156
Sparkling Berry Cooler, 53
Sparkling Raspberry Limeade, 69
Spicy Berry Ketchup, 165
Red currants. See Currants, red
Riboflavin (vitamin B2), 9, 13, 33, 41
Rice, in Black Rice Bowl, 100–101
S
Salad dressings
Berry Salad Dressing Blueprint, 120
Creamy Acai Dressing, 100
Goji Strawberry Vinaigrette Dressing, 98
Golden Berry Salad Dressing, 99
Mulberry Salad Dressing, 97
Tangy Cranberry Dressing, 98
Salads (main dish with *), 94–96
Alpha Omega Salad*, 94–95
Autumn Salad*, 96–97
Berry Main-Dish Salad Blueprint*, 119–120
Berry Side-Dish Salad Blueprint, 120
Multi-Berry Luncheon Salad*, 96
Superfood Salad*, 95
Sandwiches. See Wraps and sandwiches
Sauces and condiments. See also Salad dressings; Syrups
about: berry dinner sauces, 132–134; low-sugar jams recipe, 85; making apple or pear sauce, 131
Berry Hummus, 172
Berry Salsa, 171
Black Currant Sauce, 132–133
Blackberry Mustard, 164
Blueberry and Tomato Salsa, 170
Blueberry Barbecue Sauce, 166–167
Blueberry Chutney, 167
Cranberry Relish, 168

Cranberry Salsa with Cilantro and Chiles, 170–171
Cranberry-White Bean Hummus, 172
Easy Curry-Berry Ketchup, 164
Elderberry Sauce, 132
Gooseberry Sauce, 134
Lingonberry Sauce, 133
Mango Goji Avocado Salsa, 169
Raspberry-Mango Relish, 130
Red Berry Guacamole, 173
Red Currant & Rosemary Chutney, 168
Red Currant Sauce, 134
Spicy Berry Ketchup, 165
Strawberry Barbecue Sauce, 166
Sweet & Sour Black Currant Sauce, 163–164
Scrub, blackberry, 122
Selenium, 13, 33
Sexual health, men's, 34, 80
Side dishes. See Grain sides; Veggie sides
Skin care
Berry Coconut Age-Fighting Mask, 127
Blackberry Scrub for Face & Body, 122
Blueberry Turmeric Acne Mask, 149
Gooseberry Papaya Face Pack, 141
Mulberry Face Pack, 156
Raspberry Wrinkle Softener, 155
Smoothies, 57
Snacks, 107–117
about: gelatin theme variations, 114; personalizing pops, 116
Berry Bombs, 109–110
Coconut Berry Pops, 116
Coconut Water Berry Pops, 117
DIY Cranberry Raw Food Bars, 108
Fruit-Only Leather, 111–112
Fruity Chia Pops, 115
Fruity Nut Butter Pops, 117
Homemade Vegan Blueberry Granola Bars, 110–111
No-Bake Blueberry-Coconut Bars, 107
Nut-Free Protein Bites, 109
Strawberry and Almond Fruit Roll-Ups, 113–114
Super Berry Fruit Leather, 112–113
Whole Berry Gelatin, 106, 114–115
Soup, dessert, 144
Soups and stews, 89–94
about: cumin benefits in, 90; starter soups, 121–122
All Things Red Gazpacho, 121
Cucumber and Gooseberry Soup, 93–94
Edamame Strawberry Stew, 125
Goji Berry Soup, 122
Quinoa Cranberry Red Soup, 92

Raspberry Buffalo Slow Cooker Chili, 89–90
Red Currant Cocoa Stew, 91
Spicy Strawberry Gazpacho, 121
Squash in dishes, 96–97, 126, 139
Storing berries. See specific berries
Strawberries, 48–51
about: buying, 50; general information, 50–51, 165, 175; health-supporting role, 49–50; improving taste of, 50; nutrition profile, 48–49; storing, 50–51; things to be aware of, 51; using/uses, 51
All Things Red Gazpacho, 121
Avocado-Bean-Berry Sandwich, 104
Berry-Infused Iced Green Tea, 67
Berry Sangria, 71
Berry Shortcake Biscuits, 149–150
Chocolate-Dipped Strawberries, 160
Edamame Strawberry Stew, 125
Fruit-Only Leather, 111–112
Fruity Nut Butter Pops, 117
Fruity Salmon, 131
Goji Strawberry Vinaigrette Dressing, 98
Morning Glory Juice, 60
Multi-Berry Luncheon Salad, 96
Paleo-Style Strawberry Pancakes, 77
Red Berry Guacamole, 173
Red Cobbler, 156
Spicy Strawberry Gazpacho, 121
Strawberry and Almond Fruit Roll-Ups, 113–114
Strawberry Barbecue Sauce, 166
Strawberry Basil Soda, 55
Strawberry Chia Pudding, 86
Strawberry-Rosé Spritzer, 72
Strep throat, 22
Superfood Salad, 95
Sweet potatoes, mashed with berries, 138–139
Sweet potatoes, smothered, 123
Sweets. See Desserts; Snacks
Syrups
about: maple, nutritional benefits, 113
Berry Breakfast Syrup, 78
Elderberry Syrup, 62–63
Homemade Berry Syrup, 58
T
Teas, 61–67
about: cold, 66–67; hot, 61–64
Berry Herbal Tea with Orange Spices, 65
Berry Iced Tea, 67
Berry-Infused Iced Green Tea, 67
Blackberry Mint Iced Tea, 66
Goji Berry Tea, 65
Hawthorn Berry Tea, 63
Mulled Berry Tea, 64
White Berry Tea, 61

Therapeutic recipes. See also Skin care
Cranberry Drink, 62
Elderberry Syrup, 62–63
Hawthorn Berry Tea, 63
Thiamine (vitamin B1), 10, 13, 79
Turkey. See Poultry
U
Urinary tract infections (UTIs), iv, 14, 21–22, 61, 69, 93, 126, 133
Using berries. See specific berries
V
Vegetarian main dishes, 123–126
Acorn Squash with Walnuts & Cranberries, 126
Edamame Strawberry Stew, 125
Slow Cooker Berry-Bean Sloppy Joes, 118, 124
Smothered Sweet Potatoes, 123
Veggie sides, 137–141
Blackberry Green Beans, 137–138
Brussels Sprouts with Walnuts and Dried Cranberries, 141
Goji Spaghetti Squash, 139
Mashed Sweet Potatoes with Berries, 138–139
Spicy Berry Greens, 140
Vitamin A, 3, 12, 13, 30, 33, 35, 38
Vitamin B1. See Thiamine
Vitamin B2. See Riboflavin
Vitamin B5. See Pantothenic acid
Vitamin B6, 8, 30, 48, 136, 169
Vitamin B9. See Folate
Vitamin C, 8, 12–14, 17, 20, 24, 27, 30, 33, 36, 39, 41, 44, 48–49, 126, 134, 169
Vitamin E, 13, 14, 20, 44
Vitamin K, 13, 14, 17, 21, 28, 41, 44, 108, 173
Vitamins, discovery of, 3
W
Waffles, gluten free coconut-berry, 74, 77–78
Watermelon Strawberry Sipper, 68
Weight loss, 28, 31
Well-being, overall, 33
Wine, drinks with. See Cocktails and mocktails
Wraps and sandwiches, 103–105
about: berry sandwich ideas, 105
Avocado-Bean-Berry Sandwich, 104
Berry Nut Butter Pocket, 103
Blueberry Chicken Salad Sandwich, 104–105
Blueberry Sliders, 127
Pulled Pork Surprise Wrap, 105
Slow Cooker Berry-Bean Sloppy Joes, 118, 124
Y
Youthfulness, maintaining, 18
Z
Zinc, 10, 13, 111, 170

MAD LIBS®

Fear factor

Ultimate Gross Out!

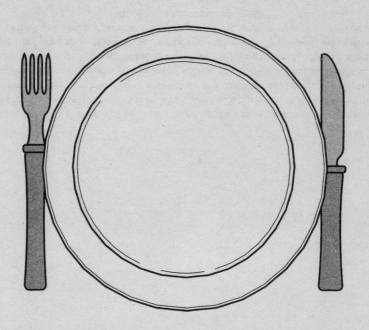

By Roger Price and Leonard Stern

PSS!
PRICE STERN SLOAN

Mad Libs format copyright © 2004 by Price Stern Sloan.
All rights reserved.
Published by Price Stern Sloan, a division of Penguin Young Readers Group,
345 Hudson Street, New York, NY 10014.

Based on the television show *Fear Factor*™ & © 2004 NBC, Inc.
under license from Endemol USA Inc.

ISBN 0-8431-1157-7

1 3 5 7 9 10 8 6 4 2

PSS! and *MAD LIBS* are registered trademarks of Penguin Group (USA) Inc.

MAD LIBS®
QUICK REVIEW

In case you have forgotten what adjectives, adverbs, nouns, and verbs are, here is a quick review:

An ADJECTIVE describes something or somebody. *Lumpy, soft, ugly, messy,* and *short* are adjectives.

An ADVERB tells how something is done. It modifies a verb and usually ends in "ly." *Modestly, stupidly, greedily,* and *carefully* are adverbs.

A NOUN is the name of a person, place, or thing. *Sidewalk, umbrella, bridle, bathtub,* and *nose* are nouns.

A VERB is an action word. *Run, pitch, jump,* and *swim* are verbs. Put the verbs in past tense if the directions say PAST TENSE. *Ran, pitched, jumped,* and *swam* are verbs in the past tense.

When we ask for A PLACE, we mean any sort of place: a country or city *(Spain, Cleveland)* or a room *(bathroom, kitchen).*

An EXCLAMATION or SILLY WORD is any sort of funny sound, gasp, grunt, or outcry, like *Wow!, Ouch!, Whomp!, Ick!,* and *Gadzooks!*

When we ask for specific words, like a NUMBER, a COLOR, an ANIMAL, or a PART OF THE BODY, we mean a word that is one of those things, like *seven, blue, horse,* or *head.*

When we ask for a PLURAL, it means more than one. For example, *cat* pluralized is *cats.*

MAD LIBS® is fun to play with friends, but you can also play it by yourself! To begin with, DO NOT look at the story on the page below. Fill in the blanks on this page with the words called for. Then, using the words you have selected, fill in the blank spaces in the story.

Now you've created your own hilarious MAD LIBS® game!

TO FEAR OR NOT TO FEAR

VERB _____

PLURAL NOUN _____

SOMETHING ALIVE _____

ANIMAL (PLURAL) _____

VERB _____

ADJECTIVE _____

NOUN _____

TYPE OF LIQUID _____

SOMETHING ALIVE (PLURAL) _____

VERB _____

VERB _____

ADJECTIVE _____

ADJECTIVE _____

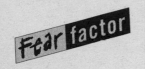

MAD LIBS
TO FEAR OR NOT TO FEAR

Hang on tight, because you're about to __Clean__ the
VERB

most disgusting _____ around! Whether you're
PLURAL NOUN

eating a giant _____ or being buried in live
SOMETHING ALIVE

_____, you'll be having some serious *Fear Factor*
ANIMAL (PLURAL)

fun! On the show, players race to _____ the grossest
VERB

things you've ever seen. Every episode brings something

_____ and new, like diving into a/an
ADJECTIVE

_____ full of dirty _____ or putting
NOUN TYPE OF LIQUID

wiggling _____ into your mouth. You'll have to
SOMETHING ALIVE (PLURAL)

_____ weird animals and _____ _____ body
VERB VERB ADJECTIVE

parts. One thing's for sure: If you can do these _____
ADJECTIVE

stunts, fear is not a factor for you!

From *Fear Factor™ Mad Libs®: Ultimate Gross Out!* Based on the television show *Fear Factor™* & © 2004
NBC, Inc. under license from Endemol USA Inc. • Copyright © 2004 by Price Stern Sloan, a division of
Penguin Young Readers Group, 345 Hudson Street, New York, New York 10014.

MAD LIBS® is fun to play with friends, but you can also play it by yourself! To begin with, DO NOT look at the story on the page below. Fill in the blanks on this page with the words called for. Then, using the words you have selected, fill in the blank spaces in the story.

Now you've created your own hilarious MAD LIBS® game!

HAM AND EGGS

ADJECTIVE _____

VERB ENDING IN "ING" _____

TYPE OF LIQUID _____

PART OF THE BODY (PLURAL) _____

VERB ENDING IN "ING" _____

ADJECTIVE _____

ADJECTIVE _____

PLURAL NOUN _____

SOMETHING ALIVE (PLURAL) _____

ADVERB _____

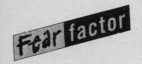

MAD LIBS
HAM AND EGGS

If you've ever been bobbing for apples, you're ready for this

_____ stunt. The only difference? Instead of apples,
    ADJECTIVE

you're _____ pig tongues, and the bucket isn't full of
    VERB ENDING IN "ING"

_____; it's full of raw ostrich eggs! Sounds delicious, right?
  TYPE OF LIQUID

The object of the stunt is to fish the tongues out using only your

teeth and _____ as fast as you can, and then eat
    PART OF THE BODY (PLURAL)

them once you've taken them out. _____ them out is
    VERB ENDING IN "ING"

hard, since you can't see in the gooey, _____ mess of
    ADJECTIVE

ostrich eggs, but eating them might be more _____: Pig
    ADJECTIVE

tongue is one of the chewiest _____ ever! Once you're
    PLURAL NOUN

done, you've got a dish of live _____ to finish off.
    SOMETHING ALIVE (PLURAL)

Take it one bite at a time, and don't eat too _____, or
    ADVERB

you might look like a pig!

MAD LIBS® is fun to play with friends, but you can also play it by yourself! To begin with, DO NOT look at the story on the page below. Fill in the blanks on this page with the words called for. Then, using the words you have selected, fill in the blank spaces in the story.

Now you've created your own hilarious MAD LIBS® game!

SQUIRMY THINGS

NOUN _____

ADJECTIVE_____

ADJECTIVE_____

SOMETHING ALIVE (PLURAL) _____

ADJECTIVE_____

PLURAL NOUN _____

COLOR_____

VERB _____

PART OF THE BODY_____

ADJECTIVE_____

VERB ENDING IN "ING" _____

ADJECTIVE_____

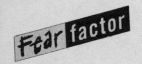

MAD LIBS
SQUIRMY THINGS

Something's squirming in that big _____ over there—
NOUN

time for some _____ *Fear Factor* fun with worms
ADJECTIVE

and snakes! When you see worms on this _____
ADJECTIVE

show, don't expect the earthworms in your backyard. Compared to

the _____ on *Fear Factor*, those are just plain fun to
SOMETHING ALIVE (PLURAL)

eat! Here we've got giant, _____ nightcrawlers,
ADJECTIVE

chewy blood-sucking leeches, wiggling _____, and foul-
PLURAL NOUN

smelling _____ worms. Make sure you _____
COLOR   VERB

the leeches thoroughly before you swallow—you don't want those

alive in your _____! And of course there's our
PART OF THE BODY

favorite worm, the wax worm. It's fat and _____ like
ADJECTIVE

a maggot, but even bigger. You might start wishing you were

_____ in snakes by the time you're done with the
VERB ENDING IN "ING"

_____ worms. Snakes are bigger and just as squirmy,
ADJECTIVE

but at least you don't have to eat them!

MAD LIBS® is fun to play with friends, but you can also play it by yourself! To begin with, DO NOT look at the story on the page below. Fill in the blanks on this page with the words called for. Then, using the words you have selected, fill in the blank spaces in the story.

Now you've created your own hilarious MAD LIBS® game!

FEAR FACTOR BILLIARDS

NUMBER _____

ADJECTIVE_____

PART OF THE BODY (PLURAL) _____

NUMBER _____

TYPE OF INSECT (PLURAL) _____

VERB _____

ADJECTIVE_____

VERB _____

COLOR_____

TYPE OF FOOD (PLURAL) _____

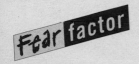

MAD LIBS
FEAR FACTOR BILLIARDS

Hope you're a good pool player! You have _____

NUMBER

shots to sink four balls, and each ball left on the table when you're

done stands for a different _____ food you have to

ADJECTIVE

eat! The options are, as always, delectable. There are Japanese

fermented squid _____ , spicy habanero peppers,

PART OF THE BODY (PLURAL)

_____-year-old duck eggs, and hundreds of tiny live

NUMBER

_____. Aim for the ball that stands for the food you

TYPE OF INSECT (PLURAL)

_____ the most, so you don't have to eat it. But

VERB

make sure the shot isn't too _____ : If you miss, that's

ADJECTIVE

one more disgusting food you have to devour. It's suggested that you

_____ for the duck eggs. They're so old that the yolks

VERB

turned _____ because they're covered in mold. I don't

COLOR

know about you, but I prefer my _____ mold-free!

TYPE OF FOOD (PLURAL)

MAD LIBS® is fun to play with friends, but you can also play it by yourself! To begin with, DO NOT look at the story on the page below. Fill in the blanks on this page with the words called for. Then, using the words you have selected, fill in the blank spaces in the story.

Now you've created your own hilarious MAD LIBS® game!

PUT UP A STINK

ADJECTIVE_____

VERB ENDING IN "ING" _____

PLURAL NOUN _____

VERB _____

NOUN _____

VERB _____

VERB _____

PART OF THE BODY _____

ADJECTIVE_____

NOUN _____

ADJECTIVE_____

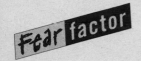

MAD LIBS
PUT UP A STINK

Something smells funny over here . . . could it be that

_____ tank full of stink beetles? Yup, that's probably
    ADJECTIVE

it! As if _____ near the beetles and smelling their
    VERB ENDING IN "ING"

lovely _____ wasn't bad enough, now you have to
    PLURAL NOUN

eat them! They're crunchy and juicy and probably the smelliest

things you will ever _____. You have to pick each
    VERB

_____ up before you eat it, then chew and swallow.
    NOUN

They might be hard to _____, since they're running
    VERB

loose and they're pretty slimy. There are two techniques you might

_____: either put them in your _____
    VERB   PART OF THE BODY

and chew them one at a time, or pick up as many as you

can and take a/an _____ bite. The second
    ADJECTIVE

_____ is faster, but be _____. They
    NOUN   ADJECTIVE

taste pretty disgusting, so you might get sick. Hopefully, you've got a

toothbrush on you!

MAD LIBS® is fun to play with friends, but you can also play it by yourself! To begin with, DO NOT look at the story on the page below. Fill in the blanks on this page with the words called for. Then, using the words you have selected, fill in the blank spaces in the story.

Now you've created your own hilarious MAD LIBS® game!

BURIED IN BEES

NUMBER _____

ADJECTIVE _____

PLURAL NOUN _____

VERB _____

ADVERB _____

ADJECTIVE _____

VERB _____

ADJECTIVE _____

NOUN _____

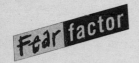

MAD LIBS
BURIED IN BEES

Bee careful . . . you might get stung! In fact, you definitely will, with

_____ bees all over your body! Twenty pounds of bees can do a
   NUMBER

lot of stinging! The bees have a/an _____ reason to
                                  ADJECTIVE

sting you, though: You're fishing around in their _____,
                                         PLURAL NOUN

looking for keys to _____ your partner's shackles.
                         VERB

Your partner is covered in even more bees, so work

_____! Bees only sting when they are upset or
      ADVERB

_____, so don't slap them or _____
    ADJECTIVE   VERB

them; it will make them even angrier. But if you take too much time,

your partner won't be too _____ either, so try to
                              ADJECTIVE

balance speed and _____. Be fast, and bee-ware!
                       NOUN

From *Fear Factor*™ *Mad Libs®: Ultimate Gross Out!* Based on the television show *Fear Factor*™ & © 2004
NBC, Inc. under license from Endemol USA Inc. • Copyright © 2004 by Price Stern Sloan, a division of
Penguin Young Readers Group, 345 Hudson Street, New York, New York 10014.

MAD LIBS® is fun to play with friends, but you can also play it by yourself! To begin with, DO NOT look at the story on the page below. Fill in the blanks on this page with the words called for. Then, using the words you have selected, fill in the blank spaces in the story.

Now you've created your own hilarious MAD LIBS® game!

WORM JUICE

ADJECTIVE _____

VERB _____

NOUN _____

VERB _____

PART OF THE BODY (PLURAL) _____

FOREIGN COUNTRY _____

NUMBER _____

ADJECTIVE _____

ADJECTIVE _____

ANIMAL _____

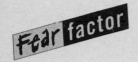

MAD LIBS
WORM JUICE

Everyone likes juice, right? Well, not this type of juice! It's not made

from delicious _____ fruit. It's squeezed right out of
ADJECTIVE

live, squirming worms! And not only do you have to

_____ this juice, you also have to make it! A big
VERB

_____ of worms is ready for you to stomp in!
NOUN

You'll have to _____ the worms with your
VERB

_____, just like the way they make grape juice in
PART OF THE BODY (PLURAL)

_____. Once you've made _____
FOREIGN COUNTRY   NUMBER

ounces of worm juice, you get a/an _____ break
ADJECTIVE

from having worms crawl around your feet. But now you have

to drink the juice! Swallow fast and consider yourself

_____: At least you didn't have to drink the juice
ADJECTIVE

from a/an _____!
ANIMAL

From *Fear Factor™ Mad Libs®: Ultimate Gross Out!* Based on the television show *Fear Factor™* & © 2004
NBC, Inc. under license from Endemol USA Inc. • Copyright © 2004 by Price Stern Sloan, a division of
Penguin Young Readers Group, 345 Hudson Street, New York, New York 10014.

MAD LIBS® is fun to play with friends, but you can also play it by yourself! To begin with, DO NOT look at the story on the page below. Fill in the blanks on this page with the words called for. Then, using the words you have selected, fill in the blank spaces in the story.

Now you've created your own hilarious MAD LIBS® game!

CONVEYOR BELT

VERB _____

NUMBER _____

ADJECTIVE_____

PART OF THE BODY (PLURAL) _____

ADJECTIVE_____

VERB _____

ADJECTIVE_____

PART OF THE BODY _____

VERB _____

ADJECTIVE_____

VERB ENDING IN "ING" _____

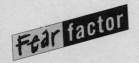

MAD LIBS
CONVEYOR BELT

So many plates, and so little time! Scoop up food off these flying

plates using only your mouth, and _____ it on a
                                              VERB

scale. First to weigh _____ ounces wins! Too bad the
                                NUMBER

_____ food is served à la *Fear Factor*! Pig
        ADJECTIVE

_____, codfish egg sacs, and blended cow snout are
PART OF THE BODY (PLURAL)

three of the _____ dishes you'll be offered. And, of
                        ADJECTIVE

course, there are huge worms that will wiggle and

_____, making it even harder for you to grab them
        VERB

off the conveyor belt. The _____ part? You can only
                                      ADJECTIVE

use your _____ to _____ them!
              PART OF THE BODY   VERB

You don't have to eat these _____ goodies, but
                                        ADJECTIVE

_____ them in your mouth and feeling them squirm
VERB ENDING IN "ING"

might be just as bad. Good luck!

MAD LIBS® is fun to play with friends, but you can also play it by yourself! To begin with, DO NOT look at the story on the page below. Fill in the blanks on this page with the words called for. Then, using the words you have selected, fill in the blank spaces in the story.

Now you've created your own hilarious MAD LIBS® game!

MAGGOT MADNESS

ADJECTIVE_____

PLURAL NOUN _____

VERB _____

NOUN _____

PART OF THE BODY_____

VERB _____

NOUN _____

ADJECTIVE_____

VERB _____

EXCLAMATION_____

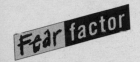

MAD LIBS
MAGGOT MADNESS

Combine three of the most _____ and disgusting

ADJECTIVE

_____ there are—cow hooves, cod-liver oil,

PLURAL NOUN

and maggots—and you wind up with this stunt. First, _____

VERB

your goggles on and dunk your _____ into a tank of

NOUN

cod-liver oil, and go bobbing for cow hooves. But you can only pick

them up with your _____! _____ in

PART OF THE BODY VERB

the murky oil for the hooves, and when you've got them, you have to

transfer them to a big _____ of _____

NOUN ADJECTIVE

maggots. Just when you drop the cow hoof, it's time to pick up a

mouthful of maggots! Put the maggots on a scale, then

_____ again—when you have enough weight, you're

VERB

done. _____!

EXCLAMATION

From *Fear Factor*™ *Mad Libs*®: *Ultimate Gross Out!* Based on the television show *Fear Factor*™ & © 2004
NBC, Inc. under license from Endemol USA Inc. • Copyright © 2004 by Price Stern Sloan, a division of
Penguin Young Readers Group, 345 Hudson Street, New York, New York 10014.

MAD LIBS® is fun to play with friends, but you can also play it by yourself! To begin with, DO NOT look at the story on the page below. Fill in the blanks on this page with the words called for. Then, using the words you have selected, fill in the blank spaces in the story.

Now you've created your own hilarious MAD LIBS® game!

EYE SEE YOU

ADJECTIVE_____

ANIMAL (PLURAL) _____

NOUN _____

ADJECTIVE_____

ANIMAL _____

TYPE OF LIQUID _____

ADVERB_____

TYPE OF FOOD (PLURAL) _____

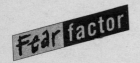

MAD LIBS
EYE SEE YOU

On *Fear Factor*, eyes are useful for lots of _____

<u>ADJECTIVE</u>

things. They're good for seeing disgusting _____

<u>ANIMAL (PLURAL)</u>

crawling all over you, they're good for closing when you're on a high

_____ and are too scared to look down—and, of

<u>NOUN</u>

course, they're good for eating! Three of the most

_____ types of eyes on *Fear Factor* are cow, sheep,

<u>ADJECTIVE</u>

and _____ eyes. All of them are big and juicy, and

<u>ANIMAL</u>

make a big explosion of _____ when you bite down

<u>TYPE OF LIQUID</u>

_____ into them. The texture is kind of like Jell-O

<u>ADVERB</u>

and a little like _____. After this stunt, you'll be

<u>TYPE OF FOOD (PLURAL)</u>

seeing eyes in a whole new way!

From *Fear Factor™ Mad Libs®: Ultimate Gross Out!* Based on the television show *Fear Factor™* & © 2004
NBC, Inc. under license from Endemol USA Inc. • Copyright © 2004 by Price Stern Sloan, a division of
Penguin Young Readers Group, 345 Hudson Street, New York, New York 10014.

MAD LIBS® is fun to play with friends, but you can also play it by yourself! To begin with, DO NOT look at the story on the page below. Fill in the blanks on this page with the words called for. Then, using the words you have selected, fill in the blank spaces in the story.

Now you've created your own hilarious MAD LIBS® game!

A HISS GOOD-BYE

ADJECTIVE _____

VERB _____

PART OF THE BODY (PLURAL) _____

VERB (PAST TENSE) _____

FOREIGN COUNTRY _____

NUMBER _____

VERB _____

PART OF THE BODY _____

VERB _____

SOMETHING ALIVE (PLURAL) _____

NOUN _____

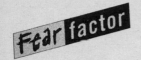

MAD LIBS
A HISS GOOD-BYE

Imagine lying in a/an _____ coffin and trying
ADJECTIVE

to _____ a pair of handcuffs off of your
VERB

_____. Sounds hard, right? Now imagine doing it
PART OF THE BODY (PLURAL)

with huge, hissing cockroaches climbing all over you! The roaches

are _____ directly from _____ for
VERB (PAST TENSE)   FOREIGN COUNTRY

this stunt. _____ of them are poured all over you in
NUMBER

your coffin to tickle, bite, and _____ you as you
VERB

try to unfasten your cuffs. You'll have goggles on so they can't

get in your _____, but they're free to
PART OF THE BODY

_____ anywhere else they want! Not only are the
VERB

cockroaches hissing and nibbling on you, they also smell like

dead _____! So be sure to bring a/an
SOMETHING ALIVE (PLURAL)

_____ for your nose!
NOUN

From *Fear Factor*™ *Mad Libs*®: *Ultimate Gross Out!* Based on the television show *Fear Factor*™ & © 2004
NBC, Inc. under license from Endemol USA Inc. • Copyright © 2004 by Price Stern Sloan, a division of
Penguin Young Readers Group, 345 Hudson Street, New York, New York 10014.

MAD LIBS® is fun to play with friends, but you can also play it by yourself! To begin with, DO NOT look at the story on the page below. Fill in the blanks on this page with the words called for. Then, using the words you have selected, fill in the blank spaces in the story.

Now you've created your own hilarious MAD LIBS® game!

SNAKE PIT

ADJECTIVE _____

NUMBER _____

ADJECTIVE _____

VERB _____

ADJECTIVE _____

NOUN _____

VERB ENDING IN "ING" _____

ADVERB _____

VERB _____

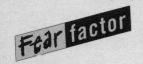

MAD LIBS
SNAKE PIT

Do I hear a hiss? That's not a Madagascar hissing cockroach, is it?

No—it's a boa constrictor! Boas and pythons will literally be

wrapped around you in this _____ stunt. On *Fear*

ADJECTIVE

Factor, the Snake Pit has some serious snakes. The shortest ones are

_____ feet long, and the _____ ones can be

NUMBER ADJECTIVE

sixteen feet in length! Sixteen feet times twenty-four snakes:

_____ your calculator, because that's three hundred

VERB

and eighty-four _____ feet of scaly snakes! You

ADJECTIVE

have to lie in a dark _____ with the snakes squirming and

NOUN

_____ around you. Move _____. The

VERB ENDING IN "ING" ADVERB

fangs of the python are famous for their ability to

_____, and you don't want any poisonous snakes

VERB

taking a bite out of you. Good luck, and happy hissing!

MAD LIBS® is fun to play with friends, but you can also play it by yourself! To begin with, DO NOT look at the story on the page below. Fill in the blanks on this page with the words called for. Then, using the words you have selected, fill in the blank spaces in the story.

Now you've created your own hilarious MAD LIBS® game!

A DREADFUL DINNER

ADJECTIVE _____

VERB _____

ADJECTIVE _____

ADVERB _____

VERB _____

VERB ENDING IN "ING" _____

PART OF THE BODY _____

VERB _____

NOUN _____

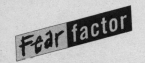

MAD LIBS
A DREADFUL DINNER

When you're going to the *Fear Factor* Restaurant, it's best to have a

strong stomach. You never know what they'll put in front of you.

Today they have two _____ selections: old, maggoty
                         ADJECTIVE

cheese and cow snout! To _____ these dishes with
                               VERB

table manners requires a/an _____ lesson in
                                   ADJECTIVE

etiquette. The cheese should be eaten _____ with
                                             ADVERB

your fingers. If the maggots start to crawl or _____
                                                      VERB

out of the cheese, ignore them and keep _____. Try
                                            VERB ENDING IN "ING"

not to breathe through your _____—smelling the
                                PART OF THE BODY

cheese might cause you to _____ all over the table!
                                VERB

The cow snout is easier to eat—just don't gag if the cow's whiskers

tickle the _____ in your throat. Take it one bite at a
                NOUN

time if you want to get through dinner *Fear Factor* style!

From *Fear Factor*™ *Mad Libs*®: *Ultimate Gross Out!* Based on the television show *Fear Factor*™ & © 2004
NBC, Inc. under license from Endemol USA Inc. • Copyright © 2004 by Price Stern Sloan, a division of
Penguin Young Readers Group, 345 Hudson Street, New York, New York 10014.

MAD LIBS® is fun to play with friends, but you can also play it by yourself! To begin with, DO NOT look at the story on the page below. Fill in the blanks on this page with the words called for. Then, using the words you have selected, fill in the blank spaces in the story.

Now you've created your own hilarious MAD LIBS® game!

OUT OF AFRICA

NUMBER _____

OCCUPATION _____

PART OF THE BODY (PLURAL) _____

ADJECTIVE_____

VERB _____

VERB ENDING IN "ING" _____

ADJECTIVE_____

ADJECTIVE_____

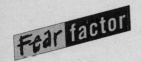

MAD LIBS
OUT OF AFRICA

Eight legs, _____ eyes, and two tiny clicking claws—
NUMBER

all in one big, hairy bite! These African cave-dwelling spiders are

truly a meal fit for a/an _____, if he or she can
OCCUPATION

swallow them! The spiders have thick hair on their

_____ and their _____ claws can
PART OF THE BODY (PLURAL)   ADJECTIVE

give you trouble, too. _____ them fast, or they might
VERB

bite you! If they snap at you while you're _____
VERB ENDING IN "ING"

them in your mouth, give them a/an _____
ADJECTIVE

crunching: Revenge can be sweet. But whatever you do, make sure

you do it fast, because this _____ appetizer won't go
ADJECTIVE

down without a fight!

MAD LIBS® is fun to play with friends, but you can also play it by yourself! To begin with, DO NOT look at the story on the page below. Fill in the blanks on this page with the words called for. Then, using the words you have selected, fill in the blank spaces in the story.

Now you've created your own hilarious MAD LIBS® game!

DON'T EGG THEM ON!

ADJECTIVE_____

ADJECTIVE_____

ANIMAL (PLURAL) _____

VERB _____

PERSON IN ROOM (FEMALE)_____

YEAR _____

NUMBER _____

ADJECTIVE_____

SAME ANIMAL (PLURAL) _____

COLOR_____

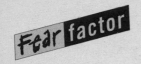

MAD LIBS
DON'T EGG THEM ON!

Fried, poached, or over-_____—however you cook
 ADJECTIVE

these eggs, they'll still be completely _____! Some
 ADJECTIVE

of the weirdest birds around, like ostriches and

_____, have laid eggs just for you to
 ANIMAL (PLURAL)

_____. We've got duck eggs that are so old and stale,
 VERB

your grandmother _____ could have eaten them for
 PERSON IN ROOM (FEMALE)

breakfast way back in _____! The ostrich eggs might not be as
 YEAR

ancient, but they make up for it by being _____
 NUMBER

times as big. It would take a/an _____ flock of
 ADJECTIVE

chickens to make an omelet this humongous! Not to mention the

eggs from the _____—those are bright
 SAME ANIMAL (PLURAL)

_____ and taste even weirder than they look! Talk
 COLOR

about an egg-stra special meal!

MAD LIBS® is fun to play with friends, but you can also play it by yourself! To begin with, DO NOT look at the story on the page below. Fill in the blanks on this page with the words called for. Then, using the words you have selected, fill in the blank spaces in the story.

Now you've created your own hilarious MAD LIBS® game!

DUMPSTER DIVE

ADJECTIVE_____

VERB _____

PLURAL NOUN _____

NOUN _____

VERB ENDING IN "ING" _____

ADVERB_____

PART OF THE BODY _____

TYPE OF LIQUID _____

NOUN _____

VERB _____

ADJECTIVE_____

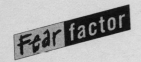

MAD LIBS
DUMPSTER DIVE

How about a refreshing, _____ dip in the pool?
                          ADJECTIVE

Wrong show! On *Fear Factor*, the only thing you'll be diving into is

a smelly, dirty dumpster! Close your eyes—it's not chlorine you will

_____, but decaying food and gross
          VERB

_____. Feel around in the _____ for
      PLURAL NOUN   NOUN

the objects you need to find: They're _____ on
                                  VERB ENDING IN "ING"

the bottom, so you'll have to search _____. And
                                         ADVERB

keep your _____ closed, because this
              PART OF THE BODY

_____ you definitely don't want to be drinking! I
    TYPE OF LIQUID

hope you remembered soap, shampoo, and _____, or
                                              NOUN

no one will want to give you a hug when you _____.
                                                VERB

You'll need a long shower to clean up from this _____
                                                  ADJECTIVE

bath!

MAD LIBS® is fun to play with friends, but you can also play it by yourself! To begin with, DO NOT look at the story on the page below. Fill in the blanks on this page with the words called for. Then, using the words you have selected, fill in the blank spaces in the story.

Now you've created your own hilarious MAD LIBS® game!

PIG IN A POKE

ADJECTIVE_____

NUMBER _____

PART OF THE BODY (PLURAL) _____

VERB _____

PART OF THE BODY _____

ADJECTIVE_____

ADJECTIVE_____

ADVERB_____

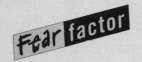

If you're expecting _____ bacon or sausage, think
                         ADJECTIVE

again. This stunt requires you to eat _____ chunks of smelly,
                                          NUMBER

rubbery pig _____. First, play a quick game of Skee-
             PART OF THE BODY (PLURAL)

Ball to _____ the amount you'll be eating. The better
               VERB

your aim, the better your stomach will be feeling pretty soon. Then

dig in! Each slab of _____ looks and smells exactly
                        PART OF THE BODY

the same: as _____ as a year-old gummy bear and as
                   ADJECTIVE

_____ as sour milk. This is one dish you won't be
      ADJECTIVE

able to eat _____, since it takes a long time to chew.
                 ADVERB

So pig out!

From *Fear Factor*™ *Mad Libs*®: *Ultimate Gross Out!* Based on the television show *Fear Factor*™ & © 2004
NBC, Inc. under license from Endemol USA Inc. • Copyright © 2004 by Price Stern Sloan, a division of
Penguin Young Readers Group, 345 Hudson Street, New York, New York 10014.

MAD LIBS® is fun to play with friends, but you can also play it by yourself! To begin with, DO NOT look at the story on the page below. Fill in the blanks on this page with the words called for. Then, using the words you have selected, fill in the blank spaces in the story.

Now you've created your own hilarious MAD LIBS® game!

SLUGS AND BILE

ADJECTIVE _____

ADJECTIVE _____

VERB _____

PART OF THE BODY _____

NOUN _____

VERB ENDING IN "ING" _____

ADJECTIVE _____

NOUN _____

ADJECTIVE _____

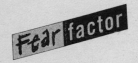

MAD LIBS
SLUGS AND BILE

Sticky as a/an _____ piece of gum, but more
                ADJECTIVE

slimy than one of the infamous *Fear Factor* superworms: you

might have some trouble getting ten of these sticky,

_____ slugs down. They're as big and greasy as they
   ADJECTIVE

come. _____ them up and put them in your
           VERB

_____ one at a time, because they might stick in
 PART OF THE BODY

your _____ if you cram in too many at once. Keep
       NOUN

chewing and swallowing—if you stop, they might start

_____ in your mouth, and that would be really
VERB ENDING IN "ING"

_____. Once you've eaten the slugs, get ready for
    ADJECTIVE

a/an _____ of cow bile. That should cleanse your
       NOUN

palate for the next _____ dish!
           ADJECTIVE

MAD LIBS® is fun to play with friends, but you can also play it by yourself! To begin with, DO NOT look at the story on the page below. Fill in the blanks on this page with the words called for. Then, using the words you have selected, fill in the blank spaces in the story.

Now you've created your own hilarious MAD LIBS® game!

THE REAL MEDUSA

NOUN _____

VERB ENDING IN "ING" _____

ADJECTIVE_____

VERB _____

PART OF THE BODY _____

SOMETHING ALIVE (PLURAL) _____

VERB _____

PART OF THE BODY (PLURAL) _____

PART OF THE BODY _____

ADVERB_____

ADJECTIVE_____

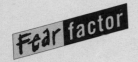
Medusa is a famous _____ in Greek mythology that
                              NOUN

can turn you to stone just by _____ at you. Her hair
                              VERB ENDING IN "ING"

is made of _____ snakes that twist and
                ADJECTIVE

_____ around her head. Now you have a chance to
      VERB

make your very own Medusa by sticking huge worms in your

_____ and spitting them out onto your partner's
  PART OF THE BODY

head! Your partner will have goggles on, so none of the slimy

_____ will _____ on their
  SOMETHING ALIVE (PLURAL)   VERB

_____, but you're stuck having them crawl all over
  PART OF THE BODY (PLURAL)

your tongue and _____. Grab a mouthful, then get
                      PART OF THE BODY

rid of them as _____ as you can. Worm breath can
                    ADVERB

be _____!
      ADJECTIVE

From *Fear Factor™ Mad Libs®: Ultimate Gross Out!* Based on the television show *Fear Factor™* & © 2004
NBC, Inc. under license from Endemol USA Inc. • Copyright © 2004 by Price Stern Sloan, a division of
Penguin Young Readers Group, 345 Hudson Street, New York, New York 10014.

MAD LIBS® is fun to play with friends, but you can also play it by yourself! To begin with, DO NOT look at the story on the page below. Fill in the blanks on this page with the words called for. Then, using the words you have selected, fill in the blank spaces in the story.

Now you've created your own hilarious MAD LIBS® game!

HOLIDAY HORRORS

ADJECTIVE_____

PLURAL NOUN _____

SOMETHING ALIVE (PLURAL) _____

ADJECTIVE_____

VERB _____

ADJECTIVE_____

ANIMAL (PLURAL) _____

VERB (PAST TENSE)_____

FOREIGN COUNTRY _____

ADJECTIVE_____

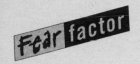

MAD LIBS
HOLIDAY HORRORS

Merry Christmas! Time to choose a gift! But this year's

_____ presents aren't the usual: Instead of

ADJECTIVE

gingerbread, toys, and _____, you'll be receiving

PLURAL NOUN

dragonflies, fermented squid coated in _____, cod

SOMETHING ALIVE (PLURAL)

sacs crawling with ants, and sausage casing containing live worms!

Pick your favorite and take a/an _____ bite.

ADJECTIVE

Whichever gift you _____, you have to eat! The

VERB

squid is as _____ as they come, the worm

ADJECTIVE

sausage is slimy and gross, and the cod sacs smell like dead

_____, so none of your choices look too good. Not

ANIMAL (PLURAL)

to mention the dragonflies, which are _____ in a

VERB (PAST TENSE)

special recipe from _____, where they are grilled

FOREIGN COUNTRY

until they are _____. This holiday season, there are

ADJECTIVE

no returns!

MAD LIBS® is fun to play with friends, but you can also play it by yourself! To begin with, DO NOT look at the story on the page below. Fill in the blanks on this page with the words called for. Then, using the words you have selected, fill in the blank spaces in the story.

Now you've created your own hilarious MAD LIBS® game!

MOO JUICE

NOUN _____

ADJECTIVE_____

PART OF THE BODY_____

VERB _____

VERB ENDING IN "ING" _____

ADJECTIVE_____

TYPE OF LIQUID _____

NUMBER _____

ADJECTIVE_____

VERB _____

ADJECTIVE_____

PLURAL NOUN _____

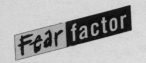

MAD LIBS
MOO JUICE

A cold _____ of moo juice is _____,
　　　　　　NOUN　　　　　　　　　　　　　　　　　　　ADJECTIVE

but we're not talking milk. In this stunt, you have to pick up cow

eyes with your _____ and pop the membranes
　　　　　　　　　PART OF THE BODY

around them, then _____ the juice inside into a
　　　　　　　　　　　　VERB

glass! Keep _____ until the glass is _____.
　　　　VERB ENDING IN "ING"　　　　　　　　　　　ADJECTIVE

If you miss, and the juice lands in your mouth, too bad. Only

_____ in the cup counts! Once your glass has
　　TYPE OF LIQUID

_____ ounces of cow-eye juice in it, take a/an
　　　NUMBER

_____ swig. You've got to _____ the
　　　ADJECTIVE　　　　　　　　　　　　　　　VERB

glass to finish the stunt. The cow eyes are squishy and

_____, and the juice isn't much better. It tastes like
　　　ADJECTIVE

old _____. Drink it fast and get it over with. Don't be
　　　PLURAL NOUN

a cow-ard!

MAD LIBS®

INSTRUCTIONS

MAD LIBS® is a game for people who don't like games!
It can be played by one, two, three, four, or forty.

• RIDICULOUSLY SIMPLE DIRECTIONS

In this tablet you will find stories containing blank spaces where words are
left out. One player, the READER, selects one of these stories. The READER
does not tell anyone what the story is about. Instead, he/she asks the other
players, the WRITERS, to give him/her words. These words are used to fill
in the blank spaces in the story.

• TO PLAY

The READER asks each WRITER in turn to call out a word—an adjective or
a noun or whatever the space calls for—and uses them to fill in the blank
spaces in the story. The result is a MAD LIBS® game.

When the READER then reads the completed MAD LIBS® game to the other
players, they will discover that they have written a story that is fantastic,
screamingly funny, shocking, silly, crazy, or just plain dumb—depending
upon which words each WRITER called out.

• EXAMPLE (*Before* and *After*)

"_____!" he said _____
         EXCLAMATION   ADVERB

as he jumped into his convertible _____ and
                                        NOUN

drove off with his _____ wife.
                          ADJECTIVE

"_____*Ouch!*_____!" he said _____*stupidly*_____
         EXCLAMATION   ADVERB

as he jumped into his convertible _____*cat*_____ and
                                        NOUN

drove off with his _____*brave*_____ wife.
                          ADJECTIVE